The Science of Smarter Kids

Thriving in the Digital Age: Building Cognitive Skills, Emotional Intelligence, and Resilience from Infancy through Adolescence

by
LEON EDWARD

Paperback ISBN: 979-8-9925482-2-8

Hardcover ISBN: 979-8-9925482-3-5

The Science of Smarter Kids

Thriving in the Digital Age: Building Cognitive Skills, Emotional Intelligence, and Resilience from Infancy through Adolescence

Contents

Chapter 1: Introduction

Embracing the journey of nurturing a child's cognitive and emotional development can be both exhilarating and daunting for parents, teachers, and caregivers. Understanding the brain's remarkable capability to grow and adapt through childhood and adolescence highlights the profound impact of our everyday choices. This book offers research-based strategies designed to support your efforts in creating environments that foster brain health and emotional resilience. As today's world presents unprecedented challenges—ranging from overstimulation to detrimental habits—it's essential to equip ourselves with the knowledge to navigate these influences effectively. By exploring each chapter, you'll find practical advice tailored to your child's age and needs, helping differentiate between essential guidance for infants to actionable tips for teenagers. Armed with this information, you play a pivotal role in shaping young minds, supporting growth, and ensuring a hopeful, balanced future.

Why Brain Health Matters at Every Stage of Childhood & Adolescence

When we talk about childhood and adolescence, it's easy to think about milestones like a baby's first steps or a teenager's high school graduation. However, beneath these visible markers, there's an intricate and dynamic process unfolding: the development of the brain. Ensuring brain health at every stage from infancy through adolescence is crucial because it lays the groundwork for cognitive abilities, emotional intelligence, and resilience to future challenges.

The human brain is a complex organ that undergoes remarkable changes during childhood and adolescence. From the rapid neural connections formed in infancy to the refining of these networks during adolescence, brain health functions as the bedrock for learning, social interactions, and emotional well-being. While each stage of development brings unique challenges and needs, prioritizing brain health in a holistic way—through nutrition, sleep, movement, and mental exercises—is essential.

Brain development begins as early as prenatal life but becomes particularly rapid during infancy and early childhood. This period is marked by the formation of billions of neural connections—akin to a fast-paced wiring of a supercomputer. During this critical window, factors such as parental care, nutritional intake, and early sensory experiences can significantly influence brain architecture (Thompson & Nelson, 2001). These early years form the base for subsequent brain maturation processes and highlight the need for a nurturing environment that promotes cognitive and emotional growth.

As children grow into school-age years, their brains continue to develop at a breathtaking pace. This stage involves the strengthening of important regions associated with language, memory, and executive functions. During these years, children benefit tremendously from mental stimulation through structured learning and play. Reading to them, encouraging exploration, and allowing free play all contribute to creating a fertile ground for learning and creativity. The interplay between genes and environment plays a pivotal role, where supportive relationships and rich experiences help solidify critical cognitive skills (Diamond & Lee, 2011).

Moving into adolescence, the brain enters a transformative phase marked by both potential and vulnerability. This period involves significant changes in the brain's prefrontal cortex, which is responsible for decision-making and impulse control. While the increased plasticity during adolescence presents opportunities for learning and adaptation, it also necessitates careful guidance to ensure that this plasticity is channeled toward positive developmental outcomes (Steinberg, 2005). Adolescents require supportive surroundings and responsible models as they navigate complex social landscapes and build their own identities.

Naturally, maintaining brain health isn't solely about cognitive development. Emotional well-being plays an equally vital role in shaping a child's or teenager's life trajectory. Stable, loving relationships with parents, teachers, and peers form the emotional scaffolding necessary for young individuals to thrive. Empathy, emotional regulation, and a positive outlook are just some of the components effectively nurtured through secure attachments. It's through these connections that children come to understand themselves and the world around them, embedding the seeds of enduring emotional intelligence (Siegel & Bryson, 2011).

The impact of a poor diet, insufficient sleep, or a lack of physical activity is often underestimated in the conversation about brain health. Simple lifestyle changes can produce profound benefits across cognitive, emotional, and physical dimensions. Nutrient-dense foods, like omega-3 fatty acids and antioxidants, provide essential building blocks for brain development (Gómez-Pinilla, 2008). Likewise, sleep remains a cornerstone in memory consolidation and emotional regulation, while physical activities promote blood flow to the brain and stimulate the growth of new neurons.

Furthermore, the digital age presents unique challenges and opportunities. Technology, when used wisely, can facilitate educational growth and enhance problem-solving skills. However, excessive screen time without the balance of physical activity and face-to-face interaction can hinder emotional and cognitive development. Thus, setting age-appropriate boundaries and teaching children how to use technology mindfully becomes fundamental in supporting their brain health.

Addressing brain health from infancy through adolescence requires a concerted and informed effort from parents, educators, and caregivers alike. Understanding the stages of brain development provides critical insights into remaining proactive and responsive to the needs of young minds. With a thoughtful combination of nutrition, adequate rest, physical activity, and emotional support, we can empower children not only to reach their full potential but to carry forward a foundation of well-being throughout their lives.

The exploration of brain health across different life stages guides us in protective and enriching practices. It's not only about enhancing cognitive capabilities or cultivating emotional resilience; it's about fostering an environment where children and teenagers can derive joy, develop empathy, and gain a profound understanding of themselves and their place in the world. As we move forward, let's prioritize brain health at each developmental milestone, enabling stronger, healthier, and happier futures for our children.

Understanding Cognitive Development and Emotional Well-being

The journey of cognitive development and emotional well-being is both complex and fascinating. From the earliest days of life, children's brains undergo rapid transformations, laying the foundation for a multitude of cognitive skills and emotional capacities. Understanding these processes is crucial for parents, teachers, and caregivers who seek to nurture children's potential in a balanced and supportive environment.

Cognitive and emotional development are deeply intertwined, each influencing the other. Cognitive skills such as memory, attention, and problem-solving provide children with the tools to interpret and engage with their world. Simultaneously, emotional well-being fuels motivation and resilience, empowering children to confront challenges and grow from them. When these aspects of development are harmonized, children are better equipped to thrive both academically and socially (Dweck, 2015).

During early childhood, the brain is at its most malleable, allowing for significant learning and adaptation. This period is marked by the formation of neural connections at a staggering rate. These first few years also establish patterns for emotional regulation and social interaction. Here, the responsive and empathetic caregiving environment plays a pivotal role. Whether it's through game-playing, storytelling, or simple attentive interaction, the quality of early experiences can significantly impact children's cognitive development and emotional health (Siegel, 2012).

As children progress into school age, their cognitive and emotional landscapes continue to evolve. School-age children begin to hone specific cognitive skills, including executive functions such as working memory, cognitive flexibility, and inhibitory control. Emotional growth is evident in their ability to form and sustain relationships, manage stress, and develop empathy. This ongoing development is not just a matter of growth but adaptation—adjusting to new information and changing environments (Giedd et al., 2009).

Nurturing this growth involves not only biological and environmental inputs but also intentional strategies. Thoughtful engagement in activities like reading, physical exercise, and structured challenges helps build cognitive capacities. Likewise, fostering a stable emotional environment, where kids feel safe to express themselves and explore feelings, can bolster emotional intelligence. Intentional practice of goal-setting, reflection, and emotional regulation strategies benefits their growth both now and in adulthood (Dweck, 2015).

Mindful nutrition, sleep hygiene, and movement are integral elements that support cognitive and emotional well-being. Diets rich in omega-3 fatty acids, antioxidants, and other essential nutrients have been shown to promote brain health. Adequate and consistent sleep patterns are crucial for cognitive functions like memory consolidation and emotional processing. Physical activities ranging from structured sports to free play are proven to enhance cognitive efficiency and emotional resilience (Siegel, 2020).

Moreover, as they mature, children need support to navigate the challenges of modern life, including digital engagement and academic pressures. Finding a healthy balance with screen time and encouraging active engagement in real-world activities is crucial. Parents and caregivers can set boundaries and guide children in making conscious choices about their media consumption and social interactions. Such balance helps prevent overstimulation and supports healthier, more regulated emotional experiences (Giedd et al., 2009).

The dynamics of cognitive development and emotional well-being also highlight the importance of community—an interconnected web of relationships that provides support, guidance, and encouragement. Schools, families, and peer groups create networks where children can practice their cognitive and emotional skills. Communities that value inclusive and supportive atmospheres help foster environments where children of all backgrounds and abilities can flourish (Dweck, 2015).

Ultimately, understanding cognitive development and emotional well-being underscores a profound yet simple truth: every child's journey is unique. Although foundational knowledge can provide a roadmap, acknowledging individual differences empowers caregivers to tailor their support to each child's needs. By fostering a nurturing, stimulating, and empathetic environment, we ensure that children are not only able to succeed in school but grow into capable, connected, and compassionate individuals.

How to Read This Book: Navigating the Chapters Based on Your Child's Age & Needs

Diving into this book, you might be wondering how to make the most of its content given your unique situation. From infants just beginning their journey to teenagers braving the complex pathways of adolescence, each stage of a child's cognitive and emotional development presents distinct needs and challenges. This book is structured to accommodate those differences, offering targeted advice, strategies, and insights that align with where your child or children are on their developmental path.

Let's start with infants and toddlers. The brain development in these early years is nothing short of remarkable. Neural connections form rapidly, laying the groundwork for future learning and emotional intelligence ("Shonkoff, 2011"). You'll find dedicated chapters on nurturing these early developmental stages with insights on nutrition, movement, and the paramount importance of attachment and love. Even the earliest interactions—those first smiles and coos—can influence brain architecture in profound ways, so we've placed a strong emphasis on how you can optimize these experiences.

For parents of preschoolers and young kids, your role shifts slightly as your child starts to explore the world with more independence. This shift requires a fine balance between providing security and encouraging curiosity. Look to chapters that address how sleep, play, and an engaging environment contribute to your child's burgeoning cognitive skills. You'll find practical advice on setting routines and choosing activities that promote brain health and emotional well-being ("Siegel, 2012").

Once they reach the school-age phase, kids are primed for learning. Academic success, emotional resilience, and physical health are increasingly intertwined during these years. Our chapters discussing nutrition and mental stimulation become particularly relevant here. Research shows the right diet can enhance cognitive performance, while mental exercises can bolster memory and problem-solving skills ("Deary et al., 2007"). By implementing the book's suggestions, you'll be equipping your child with tools they need for both academic and personal success.

Teenagers, with their complex brains undergoing further growth and refinement, need a slightly different approach. They're capable of deep reflection and are developing critical thinking skills, but they're also more susceptible to stress and peer pressure. Our sections on managing stress and balancing screen time are key here. Understanding how digital distractions and modern challenges can impact your teen's brain health will empower you to set up healthier habits and limits.

The strategies offered throughout this book apply broadly but also contain specific advice for varied stages because brain development is an ever-evolving process. Students of developmental psychology acknowledge that while foundational skills are built early, the adolescent brain is still remarkably plastic (Giedd, 2004). As a parent, teacher, or caregiver, you hold significant influence over how this plasticity is directed.

Use this book as a guide, knowing that each chapter is crafted to address the specific needs relative to your child's age and stage of development. Navigate to the chapters that resonate most with your current needs. While structure is provided, flexibility is essential to tailor the information to your circumstances. Feel empowered to dip into various sections based on emerging challenges or anticipated transitions, such as entering a new school year or dealing with the emotional ups and downs of puberty.

Ultimately, the goal is to offer a comprehensive resource that respects your unique perspective and the individual nature of every child. The knowledge contained within these pages is a blend of scientific insights and practical advice, designed to support every adult committed to nurturing the mind and heart of a developing child.

The Role of Parents, Teachers, and Caregivers in Supporting Brain Growth

Brain development is a remarkable journey that begins even before birth and continues well into young adulthood. With each new experience and interaction, children's brains grow and form intricate neural connections that will shape their future learning, behavior, and emotional health. As parents, teachers, and caregivers, understanding your pivotal role in this developmental process is crucial. Not only do you serve as the primary architects of their early experiences, but you also provide the scaffolding that supports all aspects of cognitive and emotional growth.

It might be easy to underestimate the sheer influence of your daily interactions with children, but consider this: Every word spoken, every emotion shared, and every opportunity for play offered is a stepping stone in their complex neural development (Shonkoff & Phillips, 2000). The environment you create is foundational, as it offers the sensory experiences and emotional support necessary for robust brain growth. By intentionally engaging in practices that enhance cognitive and emotional development, you are effectively laying down tracks for lifelong learning and mental well-being.

One of the most important aspects of brain growth is the nurturing of emotional intelligence. Children learn emotional regulation, empathy, and social skills largely through their interactions with significant adults. Modeling positive behavior, providing consistent emotional support, and encouraging open communication are key strategies. For instance, when children are encouraged to label their emotions, discuss how they feel, and navigate social conflicts with support, they develop crucial pathways related to emotional intelligence and social cognition (Siegel, 2012).

Equally important is the provision of a rich tapestry of experiences that challenge and stimulate young minds. Parents and caregivers can weave these experiences into everyday life by encouraging exploration and curiosity. Allow children to ask questions, experiment with new ideas, and engage in problem-solving activities. This kind of cognitive stimulation fosters higher-order thinking and creativity, as it encourages the brain to make new connections and adapt to novel situations. Teachers, too, play a critical role by designing curricula that are both challenging and supportive, catering to the diverse needs of each child (Dweck, 2006).

Your role in supporting a healthy lifestyle can't be overstated. Physical activity is essential for brain health, and parents and teachers can encourage it by promoting regular play, sports, and active learning. Exercise is not only beneficial for physical health but also for cognitive function, improving attention, problem-solving skills, and emotional resilience (Ratey & Hagerman, 2008). Ensure that children have opportunities for both structured and free play, as these activities promote creativity and emotional expression.

Nutrition is another cornerstone of brain growth, directly impacting cognitive performance and development. Parents have the responsibility to introduce brain-boosting foods rich in omega-3 fatty acids, vitamins, and minerals that support neural health. Teachers and school administrators can advocate for healthier school meal programs and educate children on the importance of a balanced diet. By incorporating these practices, you're not just nurturing the body but enhancing cognitive capacities as well (Gómez-Pinilla, 2008).

In the classroom, teachers wield the power to create an enriched learning environment that caters to the brain's need for varied stimuli. Integrating diverse teaching methods—including visual, auditory, and kinesthetic activities—ensures that children engage multiple brain regions, thereby strengthening different neural pathways. Collaborative projects, hands-on experiments, and multimedia resources can make learning both enjoyable and effective, thus promoting sustained cognitive engagement (Bransford et al., 2000).

In an age of digital distractions, managing screen time has become an integral part of supporting brain growth. Adults must be mindful of the potential negative effects of excessive screen exposure, such as reduced attention spans and impaired social skills. Balance is key. Encourage children to engage in offline activities that involve physical movement, social interaction, and creative play. Establishing healthy digital habits from a young age helps safeguard children's cognitive and emotional development (Christakis et al., 2018).

Finally, strong partnerships among parents, teachers, and caregivers are fundamental to optimizing brain growth. Consistent communication and collaboration ensure that strategies for supporting development are reinforced across different environments. Share insights, celebrate successes, and work together to address any challenges. When adults collaborate effectively, the positive impact on children is profound, creating an encompassing support system that nurtures every aspect of their brain development.

In all, understanding your role in supporting brain growth is about recognizing that every gesture, word, and decision influences a child's cognitive and emotional journey. Armed with empathy, knowledge of scientific principles, and a collaborative spirit, you can empower yourself to shape a future where children reach their fullest potential.

How This Book Can Help: Research-Based, Practical, and Real-World Strategies

As caregivers, parents, and educators, we stand on the front lines of childhood and adolescent development. The complexities of fostering a nurturing environment for the brains of our youth can't be understated. Brains brimming with potential need the right conditions to flourish, and this is where cutting-edge research, practical wisdom, and real-world strategies come into play. Our intent is to present you with insights rooted in science and crafted through experience, aimed at empowering you to support and enhance cognitive and emotional development in children.

Our journey begins by unraveling the intricate layers of brain health and its significance across various developmental stages. Each chapter distills complex research into digestible information, presenting strategies that fit seamlessly into daily life. For instance, understanding the rapid growth of neural connections during early childhood equips you to foster environments that stimulate robust brain development (Gopnik et al., 1999). This book provides insights into how love, responsive caregiving, and even simple acts like reading aloud can strengthen these neural pathways.

In parallel, we dive into essential practices that advocate brain health through nutrition, sleep, movement, and mental exercises. Nutrition, a pivotal aspect of brain health, gets a spotlight in our exploration of brain-boosting foods and their benefits across different childhood stages. Offering guidance on what to include and avoid in your child's diet, we strive to balance scientific insight with practical applications (Bryan et al., 2004). For instance, switching sugary snacks with nutrient-dense alternatives not only boosts cognitive function but also nurtures emotional resilience.

Real-world scenarios form the backbone of our approach. We comprehensively address the impacts of technology, specifically screen time and digital engagement, which have become an inescapable reality for modern families. Identifying the fine line between beneficial and excessive screen use, we propose strategies to harness technology as an ally in cognitive development without sacrificing emotional well-being. Science tells us that moderate interaction with educational content can enhance learning and memory (Anderson and Pempek, 2005).

Sleep and its profound impact on brain function and emotional health receive equal emphasis. Consistent with research from neuroscientists and sleep experts, we break down how developing a healthy sleep routine can optimize memory retention, mood regulation, and overall cognitive performance (Owens et al., 2000). Parents and caregivers are guided to create a conducive sleep environment, which in turn supports children's mental and emotional growth.

Exercise, both physical and mental, emerges as a pillar of brain health. Physical activity is linked to brain function improvements through increased blood flow and neuroplasticity, influencing attention and problem-solving abilities (Hillman et al., 2008). The book invites you to explore simple yet effective methods to integrate more movement into children's routines, from active playtime to structured exercises that cater to various ages.

Equally critical is equipping children with mental exercises that lay the groundwork for lifelong cognitive skills. From the practice of mindfulness to the embrace of complex problem-solving activities, we extend a toolkit of strategies that fortify mental resilience, creative thinking, and emotional intelligence. Cognitive exercises, like engaging with literature or learning a new instrument, fortify mental acuity and emotional depth (Green and Bavelier, 2003).

Consciously crafted to respect individual differences and family dynamics, our recommendations are adaptable. Offering a spectrum of strategies allows you to choose approaches that resonate most with your unique circumstances and philosophies. It's about finding a balance that supports your child's development effectively, without overwhelming you or them.

By weaving together research-based strategies with relatable, real-world applications, this book serves not just as a guide but as a companion on your journey. It stands to empower you with knowledge, infuse confidence in your actions, and underscore the profound influence you have on your child's developing brain. With every strategy grounded in scientific understanding, and presented with empathy, our goal is to support you in nurturing the cognitive and emotional well-being of the children you cherish.

Together, we step into a shared commitment to elevating brain health through informed, thoughtful practices. By starting with a foundation of knowledge and compassion, you can help sculpt a world where children are not only primed to survive but to thrive in every aspect of their burgeoning lives.

Chapter 2: Brain Development in Infants & Toddlers

In the early years of life, your child's brain undergoes remarkable growth and transformation, a period marked by the rapid formation of neural connections. During the first five years, the brain develops more than one million new neural connections every second, laying the crucial groundwork for cognitive and emotional growth (Shonkoff et al., 2014). The immediate environment, filled with sensory experiences and emotional interactions, significantly impacts this development. Engaging infants and toddlers with responsive caregiving—through love, attachment, and consistent interaction—can foster secure relationships and a foundation for lifelong learning. These early experiences mold the brain's architecture and have profound effects on how a child interprets and interacts with the world (Cameron et al., 2017). Empowering caregivers with knowledge about brain-boosting nutrition, sleep, and movement not only enhances development but also mitigates negative influences such as overstimulation. As you navigate this transformative phase, remember that your nurturing presence and intentional activities are key components in supporting your child's burgeoning cognitive and emotional capacities.

How the Brain Develops in the First Five Years

It's astonishing to think about the critical foundations laid in a child's brain during the first five years of life. This period is a whirlwind of development, with the brain experiencing a massive growth spurt.

During these early years, a child's brain forms more than a million neural connections every second (Center on the Developing Child, 2017). Such a rapid pace underscores the importance of understanding this stage and providing an environment rich in opportunities for positive brain developments.

In the first year, infants undergo significant changes. You might observe your baby's transition from reflexive actions to more purposeful movements. This is when sensory experiences play a crucial role in brain development. Each sight, sound, and touch is new data for the young brain, laying down neural pathways that influence cognitive and emotional growth (Hutton et al., 2015). Parents, teachers, and caregivers should create a sensory-rich environment for infants, incorporating diverse stimuli to encourage this process naturally.

As toddlers grow, their brains become hubs of activity focused on refining connections. Synaptic pruning, the process where the brain eliminates excess neurons and synapses, is in full effect. It's fascinating that this process actually strengthens the brain's ability to adapt and learn by getting rid of unnecessary pathways. This practice underscores why high-quality interactions and varied experiences are so important during these years (Shonkoff & Phillips, 2000).

Early childhood is also the prime time for the development of emotional regulation and social skills. During this period, children learn to interpret and express their emotions—the building blocks of emotional intelligence. Interacting with caregivers who respond empathetically teaches children how to manage emotions effectively. This is not just about communication; it's about shaping the very circuitry of the brain (Siegel, 2012).

Language and communication development is another cornerstone during the first five years. Children exposed to rich language environments often show superior language skills. Speaking to children, reading with them, and engaging in conversations light up many areas of the brain, particularly those responsible for processing sound and language (Gilkerson et al., 2018). Hence, fostering an environment where language is continuously practiced can have long-lasting impacts on a child's literacy and overall cognitive capabilities.

Moreover, physical movement is integral to brain development. Activities like crawling and walking are not only physical milestones but are also linked to cognitive and emotional advancements. Movement stimulates brain growth by supporting the formation and strengthening of neural networks. It's crucial for parents and caregivers to encourage activities that promote coordination and physical exploration (Pangrazi et al., 1998).

This intriguing phase of brain development can also be influenced by diet and nutrition. Essential fatty acids, iron, zinc, copper, iodine, selenium, and vitamin A are some of the critical nutrients that support brain health. Breastfeeding is one way to support these developmental needs, providing an optimal mix of nutrients that contribute to neural development (Dewey, 2001). As children grow, ensuring a balanced diet continues to support their brain's expansion and function.

Sleep is another crucial factor in brain development. During sleep, children's brains are busy processing the day's information, organizing memories, and making connections that are vital for learning and development. Establishing good sleep patterns can greatly enhance cognitive growth. Sleep is one of the silent architects of a child's brain, underscoring its importance (Mindell & Owens, 2015).

Ultimately, the experiences and interactions a child has in the first five years are foundational to their lifelong brain health. Parents, teachers, and caregivers hold the unique responsibility of shaping these formative years. Providing a nurturing environment filled with love, care, and stimulation can cultivate a child's cognitive and emotional faculties, setting them on a trajectory for success. Recognizing the power of these early interactions and environments encourages us to rethink how we support young children's development, emphasizing strategies that promote healthy brain growth and adaptability for a vibrant future.

The Rapid Growth of Neural Connections in Infancy

The first few years of life are a period of extraordinary brain activity. During infancy, a baby's brain undergoes dramatic growth, forming new neural connections at a staggering rate that lays the foundation for cognitive and emotional development. This phase, often referred to as "synaptogenesis," is when neurons forge synapses, the vital connections that facilitate communication within the brain. At its peak, a baby's brain is capable of forming more than a million neural connections every second, dictating the child's future ability to learn and adapt (Stiles & Jernigan, 2010).

Why is this rapid synaptic growth so significant? For one, it sets the stage for critical developmental milestones in cognition, language, and emotional regulation. These initial connections are not just abundant, they are also highly adaptable, a feature neuroscientists call "plasticity" (Kolb et al., 2012). This plastic nature means the brain can be molded by experiences, both positive and negative. Hence, the environment an infant is exposed to plays a crucial role in shaping their mental and emotional faculties.

Research has shown that a nurturing and stimulating environment, rich with love, secure attachments, and sensory experiences, fosters optimal brain development during this period. In contrast, deprivation or neglect during these critical years can lead to impaired neural integration and cognitive deficits (Nelson, Fox, & Zeanah, 2014). It's no exaggeration to state that the connections formed in these early years have lifelong implications on a child's ability to think, learn, and manage emotions.

The sensory inputs — what a baby sees, hears, and feels — are instrumental in guiding synaptogenesis. For instance, exposure to language and music is known to enhance linguistic capabilities and auditory processing skills. Parents and caregivers should actively engage in verbal communication with infants, as even simple babbling helps solidify the neural pathways associated with language (Kuhl, 2010).

Visual stimuli also play a key role in brain development. Bright colors, varied shapes, and facial recognition stimulate the visual cortex, contributing to an infant's visual acuity and attention span. Additionally, the sense of touch, through activities like gentle caressing or varied textures, helps infants distinguish themselves from their surroundings and enhances somatosensory processing (Field, 2010).

It's not just about the quantity of neural connections but rather the quality and strength of these synapses. In the process known as "synaptic pruning," the brain systematically eliminates weaker connections while strengthening those that are used frequently. This "use it or lose it" principle underscores the importance of consistent, quality interactions with the environment. Active synaptic pathways become more efficient, reinforcing the skills and abilities that will serve children throughout their lives.

Understanding these processes underscores why early childhood is a critical time for intervention and support. Programs targeting early childhood development now emphasize the importance of a stimulating environment, highlighting activities that promote sensory, motor, and cognitive engagement. Simple actions, like talking to a baby, reading stories, playing music, and encouraging exploration, can have profound effects on neural development. These activities provide a framework for strong, enduring neural connections that support lifelong learning and adaptability.

While genetic factors undoubtedly influence brain development, the environment has an equally compelling role in shaping an infant's neural architecture. This interplay between genes and experiences accentuates the responsibility of parents and caregivers in providing a supportive and enrichinguplifting environment. By prioritizing positive interactions and mitigating stressful or neglectful situations, adults can help optimize an infant's neural growth trajectory.

Moreover, fostering a peaceful atmosphere is crucial as excessive stress can hinder neural development. Cortisol, a hormone released in response to stress, can negatively impact the formation and functioning of neural connections (Lupien et al., 2009). Traumatic or consistently stressful experiences can lead to long-term changes in brain architecture, affecting emotional regulation and cognitive functions.

Given this knowledge, public health initiatives stress the need for accessible parental education and support systems. Teaching parents about the significance of early neural development can empower them to make informed choices that enrich their child's developmental environment. Providing tools and resources, such as workshops and community support groups, can further enhance parents' ability to foster a nurturing and engaging environment for their growing child.

In summary, the rapid growth of neural connections during infancy is a crucial aspect of brain development. This formative period, marked by remarkable synaptic formations, underscores the importance of a supportive and stimulating environment. By understanding the impact of sensory experiences, caregiver interactions, and stress management, parents and caregivers can significantly influence their baby's cognitive and emotional strengths. These early efforts help establish a robust foundation that supports future learning, emotional well-being, and resilience.

How Early Experiences Shape Learning & Emotional Intelligence

From the moment a child enters the world, their brain begins an incredible journey of growth and change. Every early experience, whether subtle or significant, contributes to this developmental landscape. During the formative years of infancy and toddlerhood, the brain is bustling with activity, forming connections faster than at any other time in life. This period is a golden opportunity for shaping a child's learning abilities and emotional intelligence.

It's during these years that the brain's architecture is most malleable, allowing experiences to leave a deep imprint. The interactions infants and toddlers have with those around them help create the neural pathways that facilitate cognitive and emotional development. Sensory experiences, rich in variety and consistency, play a pivotal role in cultivating both intelligence and emotional well-being. When children explore their world—a smile from a parent, the sound of a lullaby, or the touch of a plush toy—they are doing more than simply taking it in; they are wiring their brain for a lifetime of learning.

A nurturing and responsive environment is essential for this process. Research shows that consistent caregiving, one where infants' needs are promptly and lovingly addressed, fosters secure attachments. These attachments become the foundation for emotional intelligence, where children learn how to interpret emotions and respond appropriately (Ainsworth et al., 1978). The development of these skills is not simply about managing personal feelings, but also about understanding and interacting with others.

The influence of early experiences can also be observed in how children learn. Cognitive flexibility, the ability to adapt to new situations or perspectives, starts early. As babies engage in play, whether reaching for a mobile or grasping at colorful building blocks, they are exercising key cognitive skills. These seemingly simple acts encourage problem-solving abilities, support memory development, and build attention spans. Over time, these foundational skills transform a child's ability to learn in more structured settings, such as school.

The home environment and the behaviors children witness also contribute to learning and emotional development. For example, caregivers who read to their children not only build language skills but also teach emotional nuances. The tales of courage, kindness, and empathy found in children's books provide lessons that extend beyond literacy (Bus et al., 1995). These stories present scenarios where children can see emotions in context, which helps them understand and express their own feelings.

Moreover, interactions with peers and non-parental adults introduce another layer of complexity to emotional development. These interactions involve sharing, negotiating, and even coping with disappointment. Each of these experiences teaches children about social dynamics and fosters emotional intelligence. Learning how to manage interactions outside the family unit prepares children for the broader social interactions of the world.

Despite their incredible potential for positive growth, early experiences can also present challenges. Environments high in stress can impact the brain's architecture, making children more susceptible to emotional difficulties. It's crucial for caregivers to manage stress levels, both their own and their children's, to mitigate these effects. Strategies like creating predictable routines and providing emotional support can buffer the negative impacts of stress (Shonkoff et al., 2012).

The role of language in shaping early learning cannot be overstated. Infants are attuned to the voices of their caregivers, and the words they hear help structure their cognitive architecture. Talking to babies about everyday activities, naming objects, and expressing sentiments enriches their vocabulary and enhances their ability to navigate the world. This early exposure expands their neural networks, making future language acquisition more seamless.

Similarly, music and rhythm contribute to early brain development, offering a joyful and effective means of learning. Singing nursery rhymes or clapping along to simple rhythms aids in developing auditory discrimination, memorization, and pattern recognition. All of these elements are crucial not only for music appreciation but also for complex cognitive tasks like mathematics and logical reasoning.

Emotionally, music has the power to soothe and regulate. Babies respond to the calmness of a lullaby or the upbeat tempo of a playful tune, often reflecting these rhythms in their mood and behavior. This interaction with music helps children learn to manage their emotions and can set a positive tone for emotional experiences.

As caregivers, the examples set for emotional regulation and expression are vital. Children absorb and mimic adult behaviors, learning how to respond to situations based on observed responses. Demonstrating calmness in the face of frustration and voicing emotions openly encourages children to adopt similar practices. It's through these modeled behaviors that children learn essential emotional management skills.

Of course, every child is unique, and the impact of early experiences can vary widely. While some children may excel with a direct, focused approach, others might thrive with more freedom to explore and experiment. Acknowledging and respecting these individual differences allows caregivers to tailor experiences that meet each child's needs, ensuring that both cognitive and emotional development are addressed.

In essence, the early years are a time of enchantment, where the foundations for lifelong learning and emotional intelligence are laid. Whether through day-to-day interactions or through purposeful activities, every moment is an opportunity to shape and enrich a child's developmental journey. By providing a supportive, engaging environment, caregivers can help unlock the immense potential that lies within every young mind.

The Role of Attachment, Love, and Responsive Caregiving

From the very moment infants open their eyes to the world, they embark on an incredible journey of brain development. During this formative period, the relationships they form play a pivotal role in shaping their neural architecture. Attachment, love, and responsive caregiving form the bedrock of this developmental stage, influencing both cognitive capabilities and emotional resilience. Understanding the significance of these elements allows parents and caregivers to create environments that foster healthy brain growth.

The first few years of life are marked by extraordinary brain growth. Synapses form at astonishing rates as infants interact with their surroundings (Shonkoff & Phillips, 2000). But it's not merely the quantity of neural connections that matters; it's the quality of emotions and interactions that sculpt these pathways. Attachment theory, a foundational concept in psychology, elucidates how infants rely on caregivers for safety and comfort. Secure attachment creates a haven from which children can explore and learn, knowing they have a reliable base to return to (Bowlby, 1988).

A strong attachment bond emboldens children to engage with their environment more confidently. Consider the various experiments showing that securely attached infants tend to demonstrate more curiosity and willingness to explore new stimuli (Ainsworth et al., 1978). These interactions feed directly into the brain's growth and adaptability—a process known as neuroplasticity. When children feel loved and secure, they're more likely to take risks in learning and develop crucial cognitive skills.

Love isn't just a feeling; it's a series of actions that nurture an infant's developing brain. Eye contact, cooing, and gentle touch all activate the release of oxytocin, often dubbed the "love hormone." This hormone plays a crucial role in social bonding and stress reduction (Feldman, 2007). When oxytocin is abundant, infants not only feel calm and connected but also experience chemical changes that promote healthy brain growth.

Responsive caregiving amplifies these effects by ensuring that an infant's needs are met timely and appropriately. This involves tuning in to the baby's cues and responding with consistency and warmth. Research has shown that when caregivers respond promptly to a baby's cries and cues, it teaches the child that the world is a predictable and safe place. This predictability is essential for emotional regulation and stress response (Tronick, 2007). Over time, children internalize these responses, leading to better self-control and emotional intelligence.

Emotional regulation, a cornerstone of emotional intelligence, can be significantly influenced by early caregiving. When caregivers model calmness and emotional attunement, infants learn to navigate their feelings with a similar sense of composure. This doesn't just contribute to individual well-being; it fosters skills essential for lifelong learning and relationships. Emotional intelligence also underpins key academic and social competencies, setting children up for success in future endeavors.

While the importance of attachment and responsive caregiving is clear, the modern world presents unique challenges. For instance, some parents may wonder how to balance work and attentive caregiving. It's not about the quantity of time but the quality of interactions. Simple acts like reading together, sharing meals, and engaging in play can make a world of difference. What matters most is being fully present and creating moments of genuine connection.

The caregiving environment can also benefit from a team approach, involving other family members, teachers, and caregivers. Creating a support network ensures that infants experience continuous, nurturing interactions, even when primary caregivers are unavailable. Consistency across different caregivers reinforces the child's understanding of love and security, which boosts their confidence and willingness to explore.

Though the emotional and social aspects are poignant, it's also critical to mention the role of genetics and biology. While each child's temperament and potential are, in part, genetically determined, the caregiving environment can either enhance or hinder the expression of their innate abilities (Shonkoff & Phillips, 2000). In other words, love and responsive caregiving can significantly optimize the child's developmental trajectory, allowing them to reach their full potential.

Considering all these factors, it's essential to recognize that attachment, love, and responsive caregiving are not just components of infancy; they set the stage for later development. The skills learned in these foundational years, such as emotional regulation and social competence, are the building blocks for later educational achievements and interpersonal relationships. Thus, parents and caregivers have an incredibly vital role in these early stages of life.

In summary, the role of attachment, love, and responsive caregiving is indispensable in the realm of brain development for infants and toddlers. These early interactions lay the groundwork for cognitive and emotional competence, setting the stage for a lifetime of learning and growth. As we uncover the intricate ways in which infants' brains develop, let us emphasize the power of love and responsive care, fostering environments that nurture the burgeoning minds and hearts of the youngest among us.

Key Foundations for Infant & Toddler Brain Health

Understanding the fundamental underpinnings of infant and toddler brain health can set the stage for optimal cognitive and emotional development. These early years, typically defined as birth to age three, are foundational. This is when the brain undergoes its most intense period of growth. Every experience, whether it's a simple touch or a complex emotional exchange, can influence the nascent architecture of the brain. Let's delve into the key factors that lay a robust foundation for brain health during this critical phase.

Nutrition is pivotal at this stage. During infancy and toddlerhood, children require a diet rich in essential fats, proteins, and micronutrients to support brain development. According to the American Academy of Pediatrics, nutrients like omega-3 fatty acids, iron, and choline play a critical role in brain health (AAP, 2021). They are essential for the formation of the myelin sheath, a protective covering around nerve fibers that boosts the efficiency of neural communication. Breastfeeding is recommended as it provides many of these nutrients in an optimal balance, fostering not just physical growth but also cognitive development.

Sleep is another cornerstone of healthy brain development. Quality sleep supports memory consolidation and emotional regulation. Young children have unique sleep needs that differ from older kids and adults. The National Sleep Foundation suggests that infants require 14-17 hours, while toddlers need 11-14 hours of sleep daily (Hirshkowitz et al., 2015). Observing and supporting proper sleep patterns helps strengthen neural connections, which is crucial as nearly 90% of a child's brain development happens by age five.

The power of movement can't be overlooked either. Movement isn't just about physical development; it's integral to brain development too. Activities like tummy time, crawling, and other motor skills encourage the growth of the cerebellum, the brain region that's vital for motor control and cognitive functions. Movement stimulates the vestibular system, enhancing balance and spatial awareness, which are essential for overall sensory integration (Hadders-Algra, 2005). As toddlers engage in more complex movements, they build neural pathways that support cognitive tasks such as problem-solving and decision-making.

Let's also consider the profound impact of responsive caregiving. Babies and toddlers thrive in environments laden with love and security. This emotional security is built through attachment, a critical bond established from the moment they arrive in the world. Utilizing loving interactions and attentive care, caregivers provide an environment where neural networks related to social skills and emotional control can flourish. Research in the field of developmental psychology demonstrates that securely attached children tend to have better social and academic outcomes (Thompson, 2016).

Another important aspect is early sensory stimulation, which includes exposure to varied sights, sounds, and tactile experiences. These stimuli are enriched by verbal interactions. Regularly talking to and reading to young children not only improves language acquisition but also stimulates areas in the brain associated with processing and understanding speech (Hart & Risley, 1995). It is vital to harness these rich, everyday interactions because they contribute significantly to linguistic and cognitive development.

It's essential to note the potential negative impacts of overstimulation. In an era where electronic devices are ubiquitous, it's crucial to strike a balance between beneficial sensory experiences and overwhelming inputs. Excessive screen time can interfere with sleep, hinder social interactions, and negatively impact brain development. As proposed by the American Academy of Pediatrics, it is advisable to limit the screen time of children under two years and instead encourage play and human interactions (AAP, 2016).

The surrounding environment is a final touchpoint worth exploring. It ought to be as rich as it is safe, allowing exploration under vigilant guidance. The environment in which a child grows can significantly impact brain development. A nurturing environment should encourage exploration and play while minimizing stressors. Stress, particularly chronic stress, can negatively impact the developing brain, leading to issues with learning and emotional regulation (Shonkoff et al., 2012).

In conclusion, the early years provide a window of opportunity like no other. By focusing on nutrition, sleep, movement, sensory experiences, and responsive caregiving, we can ensure that infants and toddlers build a solid foundation for a healthy brain. This foundation not only supports their present wellbeing but sets the precedent for future academic, social, and emotional success. While challenges will inevitably arise, understanding these key elements empowers parents, teachers, and caregivers to facilitate an environment conducive to healthy brain development.

The Role of Breastfeeding & Infant Nutrition in Brain Development

Breastfeeding is often heralded as one of the most important initial acts a parent can perform to support their infant's health, and it's deeply connected to brain development. The benefits of breastfeeding extend beyond mere bonding; they play a critical role in the complex process of brain development. Human milk is uniquely tailored to meet an infant's nutritional needs, providing a perfect balance of fats, proteins, and carbohydrates, along with vital minerals and vitamins, to fuel brain growth and development (Victora et al., 2016).

During the first few years of life, an infant's brain is growing at an astonishing rate. This is when synaptic pruning takes place, where the brain refines itself by strengthening frequently-used neural connections and discarding those less used. Breastfeeding supports this by providing essential nutrients like DHA (docosahexaenoic acid), an omega-3 fatty acid crucial for the development of the central nervous system and visual acuity (Innis, 2007). These nutrients are vital for optimal synaptic connectivity and cognitive function.

One of the key reasons breastfeeding is so beneficial is its role in the formation of the myelin sheath, a fatty layer that encases nerve fibers to enhance signal transmission between neurons. The myelin sheath is heavily reliant on the lipid-rich composition of breast milk. Vitamin B12 and choline, abundant in human milk, contribute significantly to the process of myelination, thereby supporting the brain's ability to process information efficiently and effectively (Black et al., 2012).

Infant nutrition doesn't just cater to structural development in the brain. Breastfeeding offers immunological benefits by transferring antibodies from mother to child, which helps protect against infections and fosters a healthy gut microbiome. The gut-brain axis is increasingly recognized as a crucial component in developing not only the brain but also emotional health and stability (Borre et al., 2014). A well-balanced, beneficial microbial community within the gut can influence brain chemistry by producing neuroactive compounds that can have direct effects on brain function.

For those unable to breastfeed, formula can be a viable alternative, but not all formulas are created equal. It’s essential to choose formulations enriched with DHA, ARA (arachidonic acid), and other critical nutrients found naturally in breast milk. Parents should consult healthcare providers to ensure their infants receive adequate nutrition, supporting not only growth but also cognitive and emotional development.

Introducing solid foods comes next as babies grow, usually recommended around six months. The transition to solid foods presents an opportunity to introduce brain-boosting nutrients like iron, zinc, and various vitamins necessary for continued neural development. Iron, for example, is fundamental in the production of neurotransmitters and myelin, and deficiencies during infancy can lead to cognitive delays

(Lozoff et al., 2006). A child's diet during these formative years should focus on whole foods, rich in essential nutrients, to ensure their nervous system and overall health are not compromised.

The sensory experience linked to eating can play a part in brain development as well. Tasting, touching, and smelling new foods stimulate the sensors in the brain, creating new connections and facilitating pathways that are essential for later complex cognitive tasks. Moreover, introducing a variety of flavors and textures can encourage acceptance and curiosity, laying the foundation for healthy eating habits and diverse dietary preferences as they grow.

Beyond nutrition, the act of feeding itself, whether breastfeeding or bottle feeding, fosters important emotional and social connections. This routine interaction supports an infant's emotional security and cognitive development by teaching them about comfort, trust, and reliability. Parents who actively engage and communicate with their babies during feeding times also enhance language development, as exposure to varied vocabulary and sentence structures sparks early language acquisition skills.

In conclusion, it's essential to understand that feeding goes beyond fulfilling physical hunger; it plays a critical role in brain development. Proper nutrition during infancy is a foundational element in supporting the brain's rapid growth, ensuring that both physical and emotional development are given the best possible start. Establishing a solid nutritional foundation can yield lifelong benefits, setting a child on a path to reach their cognitive and emotional potential.

Parents, teachers, and caregivers should feel empowered, equipped with knowledge about the undeniable impact nutrition has on an infant's developing brain. By understanding the role of breastfeeding and infant nutrition in brain development, they can make informed choices that support and nurture their child's cognitive and emotional growth. From the very first feed, they are investing in their child's future capabilities.

Early Sensory Stimulation: Sight, Sound, Touch & Language Exposure

In the early years of life, a child's brain acts like a sponge, absorbing everything in its environment. The sensory experiences they encounter—those involving sight, sound, touch, and language—are vital in shaping their cognitive architecture. Just as muscles grow stronger with exercise, the brain develops and fortifies connections through sensory stimulation. Each interaction offers a unique opportunity to strengthen neural pathways and prepare the ground for future learning and emotional resilience.

Vision is often one of the first senses parents notice their infant engaging with, and it plays a critical role in early development. High-contrast colors like black and white can captivate a newborn's attention, as their vision is not fully developed at birth. By around 3-4 months, infants begin to see colors and focus on objects, which is why providing visually stimulating environments is crucial. Mobiles with bright colors or visually engaging items around their crib can encourage longer periods of engagement, which in turn helps strengthen vision-related neural connections (Bertenthal et al., 2014).

Sound, too, is an early babysitter, offering infants their first introduction to the world outside the womb. The rhythmic sounds of lullabies have a calming effect, helping babies relax and even improve their sleep patterns. More importantly, the auditory cortex begins to recognize patterns in speech and other sounds from birth, setting the foundation for language development. Conversations with infants, even those that seem one-sided, are essential. These interactions not only build familiarity with language but also nurture social bonds. Studies have shown that infants exposed to more speech have better language and cognitive outcomes later in life (Hart & Risley, 1995).

Touch, the first sensory system to develop in the womb, remains a vital form of communication and connection after birth. Gentle caresses, massages, and skin-to-skin contact nurture emotional security and attachment. Touch has been linked to emotional and stress regulation, evidenced by lower cortisol levels—stress hormones—in infants who experience regular physical contact. This tactile interaction supports the development of what's known as "secure attachment," a cornerstone of emotional intelligence that allows children to explore their world with confidence and curiosity (Field, 2010).

The role of language cannot be understated in early brain development. From babbles to first words, this process unfolds gradually yet remarkably. Engaging in 'parentese'—a form of speech marked by exaggerated intonation and slower tempo—catches an infant's attention and aids language processing. Although it might feel awkward to narrate your actions to an infant, doing so provides valuable exposure to the rhythm and melody of language. Reading to children, even before they can understand, promotes early literacy skills by embedding language patterns within them. Furthermore, varied vocabulary exposure during these years can significantly influence linguistic prowess in school and beyond (Kuhl, 2011).

Creating a rich sensory environment doesn't mean overwhelming your little one with nonstop stimuli. Balance is key, as overstimulation can cause stress and counteract developmental benefits. A good practice is to observe your infant's cues for engagement and fatigue. This selective tuning helps personalize the sensory experience, ensuring it remains beneficial and not burdensome. For instance, if an infant turns away or appears disinterested, it's often time for a break (Beebe et al., 2016).

Sensory development is a collaborative dance between infants and their caregivers. Infants are innately curious, and adults can facilitate this by providing a diverse array of sensory experiences. Safe opportunities for sensory play—such as finger-painting, playing with textured toys, or listening to classical music—encourage experiential learning. This type of play cultivates critical thinking and problem-solving, laying the groundwork for cognitive skills they'll use throughout life.

However, while individual sensory experiences are important, the integration of sight, sound, touch, and language plays a notable role in creating a coherent understanding of the world. Infants begin to make connections between what they see and hear, or touch and taste. For example, an infant recognizes that the feel and taste of a toy go together, or that a caregiver's voice is linked to their loving touch. Such multisensory experiences enrich what are known as "cross-modal" interactions, which facilitate broader cognitive capabilities, enhancing learning processes and emotional understanding (Goksun et al., 2015).

In conclusion, the infancy and toddler years form a critical period of transformative growth. Supporting brain development through a balanced and responsive approach to sensory experiences can provide a robust foundation for cognitive and emotional development. Each stimulating interaction or conversation might seem minor in the moment, yet cumulatively, they build a network of neural connections that bolster a child's capacity to learn and adapt. As caregivers, understanding and harnessing the power of early sensory stimulation offers us a remarkable opportunity to enrich our children's future, one sight, sound, touch, and word at a time.

Sleep Patterns & Their Role in Cognitive Growth

The journey of brain development in infants and toddlers is akin to constructing a complex, intricate web. During these formative years, sleep emerges as a cornerstone of cognitive growth, playing a critical role in shaping a child's ability to learn, remember, and process information. Yet, it's not just a question of having enough sleep—it's about the quality and structure of sleep, as well as the regularity of sleep patterns.

In infants, the brain develops at an astonishing rate, with thousands of neural connections forming every second. Sleep, particularly REM sleep, is vital during this period. REM sleep, characterized by rapid eye movements and vivid dreams, supports the consolidation of memories and the formation of neural pathways (Lozoff et al., 2007). This stage of sleep is when the brain organizes and processes information absorbed throughout the day, helping to solidify learning and cognitive functions. A disruption in this cycle can hinder memory retention and learning capabilities, which can subsequently affect cognitive development.

For toddlers, consistent sleep schedules are equally imperative. Studies show that regularity in sleep timing contributes significantly to cognitive performance (Mindell et al., 2009). Establishing a routine helps to regulate circadian rhythms, promoting not just brain development but also emotional well-being. Sleep is pivotal in aiding toddlers' ability to learn language and engage with their environment, which are essential for cognitive growth.

Understanding the sleep needs of infants and toddlers is essential for parents and caregivers looking to foster young brains. Newborns typically sleep in short bouts throughout the day and night, averaging around 14-17 hours within a 24-hour period (Hirshkowitz et al., 2015). As children grow into toddlers, their sleep consolidates into longer stretches, generally about 11-14 hours, including naps. These guidelines reflect the necessary conditions for optimal cognitive and emotional development. An understanding of these patterns helps create a supportive environment where the brain's growth can flourish.

The link between sleep and emotional regulation is no less significant. Inadequate or irregular sleep can lead to irritability, increased stress, and difficulty handling emotional challenges. Infants and toddlers who sleep well tend to exhibit more curiosity, stability in mood, and an enhanced ability to handle frustration. Emotional regulation is not just vital for social development—it feeds directly back into cognitive growth by promoting an adaptable and resilient mental state.

Parents often grapple with the challenge of establishing healthy sleep habits amidst the unpredictable nature of early childhood. Creating a sleep-conducive environment is a practical step in ensuring children benefit cognitively from quality sleep. This can involve consistent bedtime routines, such as gentle activities like reading or singing, dimming lights an hour before sleep to cue physiological cues for rest, and ensuring comfortable sleep settings with suitable temperature and noise levels.

Furthermore, understanding the connection between nutrition and sleep can foster cognitive growth. Certain nutrients, like omega-3 fatty acids, found in breast milk and infant formula, have been associated with improved sleep patterns due to their role in brain development (Makrides et al., 1995). A nutrient-rich diet, paired with a sound sleep routine, amplifies the potential for cognitive health.

However, disruptions are inevitable. Teething, illness, or changes in routine can temporarily upset sleep patterns, but recognizing that these are transient helps manage expectations. Gradually steering back to regular routines reinforces the brain's recovery and adaptive capabilities. Hyperarousal, often resulting from overstimulation or stress, can significantly delay the onset of sleep or reduce its quality. It's crucial to create a calm and predictable pre-sleep routine that limits stimulating activities such as active play or screen time before bed.

Sleep's contribution to brain development extends beyond infancy and toddlerhood, forming a lifelong foundation for cognitive and emotional health. Establishing healthy sleep patterns early on not only aids immediate memory formation and emotional regulation but also equips children with routines that support lifelong learning habits and mental health. Parents, caregivers, and educators who cultivate these habits provide a remarkable gift—one of nurturing the potential of young minds with the promise of a balanced and resilient future.

Striking a balance and adjusting strategies as the child's needs shift helps maintain the delicate interplay between sleep and brain development. Adapting to individual needs and observing cues can make all the difference in fine-tuning these critical aspects of early childhood development.

The Importance of Movement: Tummy Time, Crawling & Early Motor Skills

From the moment an infant takes their first gentle breath, a wondrous journey of growth and development begins. Among the most critical aspects of early brain development is how movement influences cognitive and emotional growth. The early motor activities that infants engage in, such as tummy time, crawling, and other foundational motor skills, are essential for a thriving mind and body.

Let's start with tummy time. This simple activity involves placing an infant on their stomach for short periods each day. Although it might seem straightforward, tummy time helps develop neck, shoulder, arm, and back muscles, which are foundational for future motor skills. Pediatricians recommend incorporating tummy time into a baby's daily routine almost as soon as they're born. It not only reduces the risk of plagiocephaly, a condition characterized by a flat head, but also promotes neural connections critical for movement and coordination (American Academy of Pediatrics, 2018).

Crawling, often seen as the next milestone after mastering tummy time, is another significant phase in early childhood development. While some babies might skip this stage and go straight to walking, crawling offers a plethora of developmental benefits. Crawling involves the coordination of hands, knees, and feet, engaging both sides of the body and thus nurturing the development of the corpus callosum. This part of the brain facilitates communication between the two hemispheres, which is crucial for tasks ranging from reading to complex problem solving (Gieysztor et al., 2018).

Besides building strength and coordination, crawling plays a vital role in developing spatial awareness. As infants navigate their environment on all fours, they're gaining a mental map of their surroundings. This spatial recognition is foundational for later skills, such as mathematical reasoning and object manipulation. Additionally, the up-and-down, back-and-forth motion required in crawling aids in developing the vestibular system, which is responsible for balance and equilibrium (Berger, 2011).

One can't ignore how these motor skills directly tie to emotional and cognitive development. Movement encourages exploration, fostering curiosity—a fundamental trait that drives lifelong learning. When infants crawl towards a shiny object or to their caregiver's warm embrace, they're learning about cause and effect, distance, and the rewards of persistence. This exploration is not just physical; it's deeply cognitive, planting seeds for resilience and problem-solving.

Moreover, early motor activities are pivotal for sensory development. As infants move, they're not just building muscles—they're exposing themselves to a variety of sensory inputs. Tummy time, for instance, encourages babies to look around, touch different textures, and hear a range of sounds, all of which are critical for sensory integration. The more they move, the more they learn about how their bodies relate to the world around them (Adolph & Tamis-LeMonda, 2014).

For parents and caregivers, understanding and supporting these early stages of movement is vital. Practical steps can be easily integrated into daily routines. For example, ensuring safe, accessible spaces filled with age-appropriate toys stimulates both movement and mental engagement. Likewise, actively participating in play, such as encouraging gently or guiding movements, can significantly foster these skills.

The role of movement also extends beyond physical benefits. It plays a part in establishing emotional bonds. When caregivers engage with infants during tummy time or crawling, it's not just about guiding their physical activity—it's about creating meaningful interactions and building trust. This bond is essential for secure attachment and the emotional development of a child, laying the groundwork for future social interactions and relationships.

Scientific research continues to affirm the interconnectedness between movement and brain development. For example, a study by Gieysztor et al. (2018) found that children who engaged in more physical activity during infancy displayed enhanced cognitive performance later in life. It highlights that the earlier these movement-oriented experiences begin, the more profound their long-term impact on cognitive growth.

Acknowledging the variability in development, some children might take longer to hit these milestones. It's essential to approach these differences with understanding and patience. Encouraging incremental progress without undue stress ensures that movement becomes a joyful and rewarding journey rather than a pressurized race.

In summary, the importance of movement in infancy through activities like tummy time and crawling cannot be overstated. These early motor skills lay the critical foundation for cognitive processing, emotional growth, and social interaction. As we support our children in these early days, we equip them with the tools not just to survive but to thrive in an ever-evolving world.

By embracing and encouraging these natural movements, parents, and caregivers become active participants in their child's developmental journey, ensuring that the path taken is rich with opportunity and growth. As we've explored, when infants move, they're doing much more than advancing toward their next physical milestone—they're nurturing the budding neurons, synapses, and pathways that will one day define their potential.

Best Practices for Encouraging Cognitive & Emotional Development

In the early years of life, an infant's brain develops at a pace unmatched by any other stage of human development. This period is not merely about physical growth; it's a critical window for cognitive and emotional advancement. During this time, the foundations of language, thought processes, emotional regulation, and relational attachments are established. The environments in which infants and toddlers are immersed play a pivotal role in this intricate dance of development. Adults can significantly shape these outcomes by fostering enriching experiences that support growth holistically.

One of the most effective ways to nurture cognitive and emotional development is through responsive caregiving. This approach emphasizes the importance of responding to a child's cues and needs with sensitivity and affection. When caregivers consistently meet a child's needs, they promote a sense of security and trust, which is fundamental for healthy attachment. Secure attachment, in turn, lays down the neural pathways conducive to emotional regulation and social competence as children grow (Ainsworth & Bowlby, 1991).

Nurturing cognitive development can be both intentional and seamlessly integrated into daily routines. Language exposure is critical, even for newborns. As parents and caregivers talk, sing, and read to their babies, they're not only building language skills but also strengthening the neural connections associated with cognitive processing and memory (Hart & Risley, 1995). These interactions shouldn't feel like chores; they can be woven into everyday activities like diaper changes, meals, and bath time, making these moments enriching and enjoyable.

Providing diverse sensory experiences is another cornerstone of optimal brain development. Infants and toddlers learn about the world through their senses—sight, sound, taste, touch, and smell. By introducing varied textures, sounds, and sights, caregivers can help children develop these sensory skills. For instance, tactile exploration through safe, age-appropriate toys or safe food textures can be both delightful and educational. Sensory play is not only about sensory enhancement but also about promoting curiosity and cognitive flexibility (Elsabbagh et al., 2013).

The environment should encourage movement and exploration, which are vital for physical and cognitive development. Activities like tummy time, crawling, and eventually walking, are not just about motor skills. They are critical for brain development because they foster spatial awareness and coordination and strengthen the connection between physical movement and cognitive growth (Adolph & Franchak, 2017). Ensuring a safe space where children can freely move and explore is crucial.

Routines and consistency are also beneficial as they provide a structure that infants and toddlers can gradually understand and predict. This predictability can soothe children, making them feel secure, which is essential for emotional development. Bedtime routines, for example, are not just about preparing for sleep; they can include soothing activities that deepen emotional bonds and prepare the brain for restorative sleep, which is essential for learning and emotional regulation (Mindell & Williamson, 2018).

It's also important to be mindful of the types and levels of stimulation provided. While infants and toddlers require rich and stimulating environments, it's equally critical to balance this stimulation to avoid overwhelm. Overstimulation can lead to stress and anxiety, negatively impacting emotional well-being. Careful observation can guide caregivers in understanding each child's threshold and modifying activities accordingly.

Integrating music and play into daily life supports both emotional and cognitive development. Music engages various neural pathways, enhancing areas of the brain associated with emotional processing and memory (Trehub & Hannon, 2006). Singing lullabies or playing simple musical toys can be joyful and soothing experiences for children. Likewise, play is a child's primary way of exploring the world and testing out new ideas. Whether through imaginative play or games that involve problem-solving, play encourages cognitive flexibility, creativity, and social skills.

The role of nutrition is undeniably crucial as well. A balanced diet rich in fatty acids, vitamins, and minerals supports cognitive functions and emotional stability. While Chapter 4 will delve deeper into nutritional specifics, it's vital to acknowledge that nutrition fuels brain development. Breastfeeding and the introduction of nutrient-dense foods at the appropriate age support the growth of robust neural connections critical for both cognitive and emotional health (Georgieff, 2007).

Finally, it's essential to model and encourage emotional literacy from a young age. Children learn by observing the adults around them. Discussing feelings openly, labeling emotions, and demonstrating empathy equip children with the tools they need for emotional intelligence. Supportive discussions about emotions in response to everyday situations help children understand and manage their emotions effectively, preparing them to navigate complex social landscapes in the future.

Encouraging cognitive and emotional development in infants and toddlers doesn't require fancy programs or costly toys; it's about creating a loving, responsive environment that meets children where they are developmentally. By engaging in these best practices, adults can empower children to thrive, laying a strong foundation for lifelong learning and emotional wellness.

Talking to Your Baby: Why Early Language Exposure Matters

Long before a baby speaks their first word, their journey into language begins. This isn't just about cooing or making silly faces—it's a critical period for brain development that has long-lasting implications for cognitive and emotional growth. Early language exposure is like a duet between caregiver and child, where the back-and-forth rhythm fosters an environment rich in learning and connection.

The brain of an infant is like a sponge, rapidly forming millions of neural pathways every second. According to research, this window of opportunity is crucial as it determines the very foundation on which all future learning is built (Kuhl, 2011). During the first few years of life, the brain is exceptionally plastic, meaning it can easily adapt and learn from its surroundings. Language, with all its complexity and nuance, plays a significant role in this developmental phase.

Why does early exposure to language matter so much? Language is the primary medium through which children acquire knowledge, communicate feelings, and interact with the world. Studies have shown that children who are exposed to a rich linguistical environment tend to have extended vocabularies and better reading skills when they enter school (Hart & Risley, 1995). In other words, talking to your baby is setting the stage for academic success and emotional intelligence.

It's important to understand that it's not just the quantity of words, but the quality of interaction, that counts. Engaging in meaningful conversations, even if your baby can't respond in kind, encourages them to listen and eventually mimic the sounds. The rhythmic patterns of speech, the highs and lows in your tone, and the pauses between phrases—these are all cues that help infants begin to decipher the meaning behind words. This is the groundwork for developing literacy and cognitive abilities (Weisleder & Fernald, 2013).

Consider the simple act of reading a bedtime story. This isn't just a soothing ritual—it's an educational one too. When you sit with your child and go through the pages of a book, you're introducing them to new words, ideas, and experiences that they might not encounter in everyday life. This type of shared attention accelerates language acquisition and offers a unique opportunity for bonding and emotional growth. As children hear language in contexts that are emotionally charged and engaging, they are more likely to retain and understand new vocabulary.

It's fascinating to note that even the sounds of different languages can influence brain development. Babies who are exposed to multiple languages from an early age show a heightened awareness of linguistic structures, which can make them more adept at learning new languages later in life. This doesn't mean you have to be bilingual to give your child a leg up; merely talking and reading frequently will have a significant positive impact.

In practice, boosting language exposure can be as simple as narrating your day. Describe the things you see, the tasks you perform, and the emotions you feel. You can talk about what you're doing as you do it—whether it's folding laundry or cooking dinner. This constant stream of language offers infants examples of how words are used in different contexts and helps them form those vital connections in the brain.

Cognitive development is not the only benefit. Language exposure also fosters emotional development. Conversations are central to developing empathy and understanding of human emotions. When talking to babies, caregivers often use exaggerated facial expressions and emotional tones, helping children learn to recognize and respond to feelings long before they can articulate their own.

The reciprocal nature of communication teaches children about give-and-take, which is the core of social interaction. Even before they utter their first words, babies participate in this exchange by cooing, babbling, or using gestures. This is them practicing the dance of language, where they take a turn in the conversation, anticipating a response from the caregiver.

What about those moments of silence? They're essential too. Allowing a pause in conversation gives infants and toddlers the opportunity to process what's been said, to observe your facial expressions, and to prepare their responses, even if it's just through a giggle or sound. This reflective pause is part of the learning process; it teaches children that communication is a two-way street.

In our fast-paced world, the temptation of digital distractions is significant. However, it's crucial to prioritize real human interactions for young children. While educational programs and videos designed for babies can be beneficial, they're no substitute for real-life interaction. The richness of in-person communication—where infants can watch the nuances of facial expressions, hear the timbre of a voice, and feel the warmth of a caregiver's presence—is irreplaceable.

There's no single 'right' way to talk to your baby, but consistency and engagement are key. Together with tactile interactions like cuddling and playing, talking forms a holistic approach to nurturing a young brain. By intentionally creating an environment filled with words and conversation, you're offering your child a head start in life. You're equipping them with the tools they need not only to excel academically but to thrive emotionally.

In conclusion, the sheer power of early language exposure is profound. It's not just about speaking more words, but about meaningful, engaged interactions that lay the foundation for a lifetime of learning and emotional growth. As a parent, teacher, or caregiver, remember that every word spoken is an investment in the child's future—a future built on strong cognitive and emotional pillars.

Music, Play, and Sensory Exploration for Brain Growth

In the realm of infant and toddler development, the environment acts as a rich tapestry, woven with opportunities for learning and growth. Music, play, and sensory experiences hold a special place in nurturing this development. Engaging a child's senses through these activities not only entertains but also lays foundational pathways in the brain that support cognitive and emotional intelligence.

Music, with its melodic rhythms and harmonies, is more than just a source of joy. Research suggests that musical experiences in childhood can accelerate brain development, particularly in language acquisition and reading skills (Trainor & Hannon, 2013). The unique patterns found in music help young children recognize and process the patterns inherent in speech and text. Even before they can talk, infants are attuned to the beats and rhythms, which fosters auditory discrimination, a critical skill for language development.

There's magic in the seemingly simple act of singing lullabies or nursery rhymes to a baby. It's through these early musical interactions that neural circuits involved in sound processing are strengthened. A study conducted by Gerry, Unrau, and Trainor (2012) demonstrates that infants exposed to music lessons show enhanced brain responses to musical tones, setting a strong foundation for future musical and non-musical skills. For parents and caregivers, regularly incorporating music into daily routines—be it through listening, singing, or playing simple instruments—can serve as a powerful tool in supporting a child's overall brain growth.

In conjunction with music, play is another essential component in early brain development. Play is often described as the work of childhood, with its benefits extensively documented in developmental research. Free play, which allows children to explore and manipulate their environment, fosters creativity and problem-solving skills. The human brain thrives on novelty, and play provides just that, offering new scenarios and challenges that stimulate the brain's executive functions (Berk, 2014).

The type of play doesn't have to be elaborate. Simple activities like stacking blocks, pouring sand, or navigating through obstacle courses can significantly boost spatial awareness and coordination. This physical play strengthens motor skills and encourages toddlers to explore their movement capabilities. Importantly, such activities invite social interaction, enhancing communication skills as children learn to negotiate, share, and cooperate.

Additionally, sensory exploration is indispensable for nurturing well-rounded brain development. Infants and toddlers learn predominantly through their senses—touch, taste, sight, sound, and smell—each experience building neural connections. For instance, touching various textures stimulates the somatosensory system, enhancing fine motor skills as well as tactile perception. These sensory experiences encourage curiosity and support the development of cognitive pathways that later underpin more complex learning.

Creating a rich sensory environment doesn't require advanced tools or expensive toys. Consider using items from everyday life—a soft piece of fabric, fragrant herbs, water play, or even a mixture of textures like rice and beans can provide diverse sensory inputs. These everyday objects become instruments of learning, fostering an exploratory mindset in children.

When adults engage with children in these sensory explorations, they offer more than just supervision; they provide scaffolding that is crucial for learning. Joint attention, where both the child and the adult focus on the same object or activity, is particularly beneficial. This interaction enhances language development and social skills as the child learns to decode expressions and emotions associated with the shared experience.

The benefits of music, play, and sensory exploration extend into emotional development, too. These activities can serve as emotional outlets, providing opportunities for self-expression and regulation. Music, for instance, has been shown to reduce stress and anxiety in children. When coupled with play, it can support the development of resilience, teaching children how to cope with emotions and build emotional intelligence (Saarikallio & Erkkilä, 2007).

Moreover, engaging in regular sensory activities provides children with the opportunity to experiment and fail in a safe environment, learning from their experiences and building perseverance. This resilience is a cornerstone of a growth mindset, where children understand that effort leads to improvement—an idea central to positive cognitive and emotional development.

In closing, the effects of music, play, and sensory exploration extend far beyond momentary enjoyment. They play vital roles in brain development, offering a multifaceted approach to fostering growth across cognitive, social, and emotional domains. For parents, teachers, and caregivers, the key lies in regularly incorporating these elements into the daily lives of children, creating environments rich with opportunities for exploration and learning.

How to Build Healthy Sleep & Nutrition Habits from the Start

You've likely heard the saying, "You are what you eat," and there's no period more critical for this adage than the early years of a child's development. Nutrition and sleep are the cornerstones of a healthy brain during these formative years. While the brain of an infant or toddler is an extraordinary machine of development, constantly building new connections and shaping the foundation for a lifetime, it requires the right fuel and rest to operate optimally.

Let's start with nutrition. From the moment a child is born, proper nutrition becomes the backbone of their cognitive and emotional well-being. Breast milk is often considered the gold standard for infant nutrition due to its comprehensive blend of nutrients and protective antibodies that promote brain health (Victora et al., 2016). If breastfeeding isn't an option, don't worry—infant formulas have continuously improved to closely mimic these nutritional benefits.

As a child transitions to solid foods, the focus should shift to providing a balanced diet rich in fruits, vegetables, whole grains, and healthy fats. Essential nutrients such as omega-3 fatty acids, choline, iron, and zinc are critical for brain development and can be found in foods like fish, eggs, spinach, and legumes. A diet too high in sugar or processed foods can potentially hinder cognitive growth, making it important to introduce healthy eating patterns from the start (Nyaradi et al., 2013).

Besides nutrition, sleep is another crucial component of brain development. It might seem like the ultimate puzzle—getting an infant or toddler to follow a regular sleep pattern—but establishing good sleep habits early on is vital. Infants typically need 12-16 hours of sleep a day, while toddlers require 11-14 hours (Hirshkowitz et al., 2015). Creating a consistent routine that includes calming activities before bedtime can help set a foundation for healthy sleep habits.

Why is sleep so essential? During rest, the brain doesn't just turn off. It's a time of intense activity. Sleep supports the reorganization of neural connections, fostering learning and memory consolidation. Skimping on sleep can leave your young one irritable and emotional but, more critically, it may compromise their cognitive development. These early years are when children build the foundation for later skills like language acquisition, problem-solving, and emotional regulation.

Developing a sleep-friendly environment can drastically improve sleep quality. Considerations like a dark, quiet room and comfortable, safe sleeping arrangements can make a world of difference. Also, it's beneficial to establish bedtime routines—a bath, a story, or some soft music—as these can signal your child that it's time to slow down (Mindell et al., 2017).

As you shape these habits, consider the broader impact on family life as well. Parents and caregivers are powerful role models. Children watch and learn, so when they see adults eating meals packed with vegetables or prioritizing sleep, they'll likely imitate these behaviors. Community meal times around the dinner table become teachable moments for many life lessons, not just healthy eating.

Meanwhile, technology can be both a friend and foe in managing these habits. While apps can remind parents about meal planning or sleep schedules, screens can also be a distraction, especially for sleep routines. Limiting screen time, particularly before bed, can enhance both sleep quality and readiness for it. Blue light emitted from screens interferes with melatonin production, a hormone that promotes sleep (Chang et al., 2015). By setting limitations on technology, you pave the way for both better sleep and quality family interaction.

Building a framework for healthy sleep and nutrition might seem daunting in the beginning, but it's not about perfection. It's about consistency and adapting routines that cater to the unique rhythm of your child, while being mindful of their developing brains' needs.

Resources such as parenting classes, nutritional guides, and pediatric consultations can offer more tailored strategies that consider any specific needs or challenges your child might face.

In summary, the journey to instilling healthy sleep and nutrition habits from the start doesn't just benefit the immediate growth of infants and toddlers. It equips them with tools and disciplines that support lifelong cognitive and emotional resilience. An empowered child today can become an empowered adult tomorrow, capable of navigating the complexities of our world with a well-nourished brain and a well-rested mind.

Chapter 3: The Foundations of a Healthy Brain

The foundations of a healthy brain rest on the intricate balance of elements that either nurture or hinder its growth. From the very beginning, the brain's remarkable adaptability, known as neuroplasticity, allows it to develop through structures and connections shaped by experiences and environments (Kolb & Whishaw, 2009). Positive stimuli in the form of adequate nutrition, physical activity, mental engagement, and sufficient sleep form the building blocks of cognitive and emotional development. However, it's crucial to avoid pitfalls like overstimulation, a poor diet, and exposure to stressors which can compromise these foundations (Shonkoff et al., 2012). For parents, teachers, and caregivers, understanding these critical factors and their interplay allows for the fostering of supportive environments where children can thrive. Practical approaches can include encouraging social interactions, ensuring varied and balanced nutrition, and facilitating exposure to music and language (Lu et al., 2013). By acknowledging that each child's path is unique, our aim is to craft a nurturing framework that adapts and empowers every individual child to reach their potential.

The Science of Brain Growth & Neuroplasticity

The incredible growth and adaptability of the human brain during childhood and adolescence are nothing short of extraordinary. At this crucial stage, understanding brain growth and neuroplasticity can empower parents, teachers, and caregivers to nurture a child's cognitive and emotional development effectively. So, what exactly is neuroplasticity, and how does it relate to brain growth? Neuroplasticity refers to the brain's ability to change and adapt in response to experience, learning, and environmental influences (Kolb & Gibb, 2011). This inherent flexibility allows for the formation of new neural connections and the strengthening of existing ones, providing a foundation for ongoing learning and adaptation throughout life.

In the early years, children's brains are remarkably malleable. Rapid growth occurs as trillions of neural connections are formed, but it's crucial to understand that not all growth is predetermined. The brain's plastic nature ensures that experiences significantly shape its development, mirroring the adage, "use it or lose it" (Huttenlocher, 2002). This concept helps illustrate why a stimulating environment rich with opportunities for exploration, problem-solving, and interpersonal interaction is so vital for young children.

Consider, for example, the role of environmental enrichment. Research shows that exposing children to diverse experiences influences synaptic density and cognitive problem-solving abilities (Diamond et al., 1964). Simple activities like play, reading, and engaging conversations can all serve as catalysts for brain growth. These interactions build pathways in the brain, much like trails blazed through a dense forest, paving the way for efficient and effective communication networks.

During adolescence, the brain undergoes another intense period of growth and change. Previously formed pathways are pruned to enhance efficiency, optimizing neural networks for more complex thinking and emotional processing (Giedd et al., 1999). This period of "synaptic pruning" is guided by use—the more frequently certain pathways are activated, the stronger they become. It's no surprise, then, that nurturing activities that challenge and engage the brain are particularly significant during this phase. Incorporating activities that stimulate critical thinking, emotional intelligence, and social interaction not only enhances cognitive development but also strengthens the brain's resilience to stress and adversity.

Neuroplasticity is not solely about strengthening positive pathways; it also involves reducing negative influences that can impede brain growth. Chronic stress, exposure to negative environments, and harmful habits like poor diet and lack of sleep can all have detrimental effects on the developing brain (Lupien et al., 2009). Stress, for example, leads to the secretion of cortisol, which, in excessive amounts, can damage neural connections and impair learning. Recognizing these potential pitfalls, caregivers have a powerful opportunity to counteract negative influences with protective factors such as a balanced diet, regular physical activity, and consistent sleep patterns.

It's worth noting that the brain's plasticity remains throughout life, although it is most pronounced during childhood and adolescence. This enduring capacity for change underscores the idea that growth and adaptation are processes that continue well into adulthood, influenced continuously by life experiences. For caregivers, this knowledge highlights the importance of adopting a lifelong approach to brain health, fostering an environment where children feel supported and able to explore—and fail—without fear. Resilience, after all, is built on trying again.

The interplay of genetics and environment in shaping the brain's architecture shouldn't be overlooked. While genetics set certain parameters for growth, the environment plays a decisive role in enabling the full expression and realization of a child's potential (Greenough et al., 1987). Hence, a nurturing and stimulating environment propels brain development forward, whereas neglect and lack of stimulation may lead to subdued growth.

In building healthy, adaptable brains, collaboration is key. Parents, educators, and community members each hold a stake in preparing children for the complexities of life. It begins with creating positive, enriching environments, emphasizing varied learning experiences, and providing emotional support. Moreover, it involves learning from and adapting to the evolving landscape of scientific research on brain development and neuroplasticity, embracing innovations that support cognitive growth while cautioning against premature or unrealistic interventions.

Although the science behind brain growth and neuroplasticity is ever-evolving, its application is rooted in simple, tangible efforts. Encouraging curiosity, maintaining active lifestyles, instilling healthy habits, and fostering supportive relationships are all practical steps that wield significant influence over brain health. These efforts are not merely beneficial—they are transformational, offering children the tools they need to thrive both now and in the future.

The exploration of brain growth and neuroplasticity exemplifies a powerful truth: the potential within each child's brain is vast and remarkable. While science provides a framework for understanding, real-world application rests on the shoulders of those who care for and guide them. Through informed, thoughtful support, caregivers can shape not only smarter and healthier individuals but also emotionally resilient and capable ones—prepared to navigate the world with confidence and curiosity.

Key Factors That Support or Hinder Brain Development

Understanding what supports or hinders brain development is crucial for fostering a nurturing environment where children can thrive cognitively and emotionally. Science tells us that the brain doesn't develop in isolation but is influenced by a myriad of factors that can either propel growth or pose obstacles. Let's delve into how nutrition, sleep, sensory experiences, and social interactions can dramatically affect brain development.

Nutrition: Fueling Cognitive Growth

Nutrition plays a pivotal role in supporting brain development. Essential nutrients like omega-3 fatty acids, iron, and zinc are fundamental building blocks for a healthy brain. For example, DHA, an omega-3 fatty acid found in fish, is vital for the development of nerve cell membranes, contributing significantly to both cognitive performance and overall brain health (Rosenfeld & Nes, 2020). Parents and caregivers should prioritize incorporating these nutrients into their children's diets, whether through natural food sources or supplements.

On the flip side, poor dietary choices can impede cognitive growth. Diets high in sugar and processed foods not only contribute to obesity but are also linked to impaired cognitive flexibility and memory. A study by Nyaradi et al. (2013) suggests that children consuming a diet rich in processed foods show lower IQ scores compared to those with balanced diets. It's a stark reminder of how diet can create long-term impacts on mental acuity and learning abilities.

Sleep: The Brain's Restorative Necessity

Sleep is another cornerstone in the architecture of a developing brain. During sleep, brain cells repair themselves, and vital connections are strengthened through synaptic plasticity, which refers to the ability of synapses to strengthen or weaken over time, based primarily on activity levels (Walker, 2017). These connections are crucial for learning and memory consolidation. Inconsistent sleep patterns or sleep deprivation can disrupt this intricate process, leading to issues like impaired attention and emotional regulation.

The negative impact of poor sleep can't be overstated. Studies have shown that a lack of sleep in children is linked to problems with attention, behavior, learning, and emotional control (Owens, 2009). Thus, establishing healthy sleep routines becomes essential. Strategies such as maintaining consistent sleep schedules and creating calming pre-sleep rituals can pave the way for better sleep hygiene.

Sensory Experiences Shape Learning and Emotions

Our experiences shape us, and the brain is no exception. Early sensory input, encompassing everything from the warmth of touch to the melody of a lullaby, influences how neural pathways are formed. These pathways become the roadmap for how children learn and interpret their world. Research by Park et al. (2015) demonstrates that sensory-rich environments promote greater synaptic density, meaning a greater number of connections across neurons.

However, overstimulation poses its own set of challenges. Environments flooded with excessive noise, screens, and stimuli can overwhelm a child's developing sensory systems. This overstimulation can hamper attentional processes and, over time, lead to difficulties in concentrating and cognitive function. Striking a balance with ample playtime, structured learning, and calming downtime is key.

Social Interactions: The Human Connection

One of the most potent factors impacting brain development is the quality of social interactions children experience. From cooing infants to teenagers navigating the complexities of peer relationships, these interactions lay the groundwork for emotional intelligence and social understanding. Siegel (2012) argues that positive social engagement fosters resilience and emotional regulation skills, pivotal for navigating life's challenges.

Yet, negative or absent social experiences can hinder these developmental processes. Isolation or exposure to toxic social environments can impact the brain's ability to manage stress and emotions effectively. Purposive social engagement, full of rich, verbally and emotionally supportive conversations, forms the backbone of healthy emotional growth in children.

Exposure to Learning and Growth Mindset

The emphasis on applying a growth mindset, as coined by Dweck (2006), is invaluable in fostering a child's cognitive development. Children who are encouraged to view challenges as opportunities and learn from failures generally develop a more robust capacity for learning and adaptability. Emphasizing effort over innate ability helps lay down a foundation for lifelong learning.

To cultivate this mindset, adults should model positive attitudes towards learning and encourage children to approach tasks with curiosity and persistence. The impact is profound: children become less afraid of failure and more resilient in the face of setbacks, attributes beneficial not only for personal development but also for academic success.

These interwoven factors of nutrition, sleep, sensory experiences, and social interactions create an intricate tapestry that supports or hinders brain development. While the science points towards clear pathways for fostering optimal development, it's the tailored approach—considering each child's unique needs—that promises the most profound impact. Equipping adults with this understanding and the tools to apply it is what will ultimately empower the next generation to thrive cognitively and emotionally.

Chapter 4: Nutrition for a Healthy Mind

To nurture a child's mind, we must first nourish their body with optimal nutrition. Foods rich in omega-3 fatty acids, such as salmon and flaxseeds, play a crucial role in developing strong neural connections vital for learning and memory (Simopoulos, 2016). Moreover, zinc and iron found in lean meats and lentils are essential for maintaining focus and cognitive sharpness (Prado & Dewey, 2014). While colorful fruits and vegetables provide antioxidants that protect growing brains from oxidative stress, it's equally important to steer clear of processed foods laden with sugars and additives, which can impair mental processes and behavioral health (Gómez-Pinilla, 2008). Encouraging children to drink enough water can prevent dehydration-related cognitive decline, ensuring they perform at their best throughout the day. By integrating these nutritional strategies, caregivers can significantly contribute to their child's cognitive and emotional development, laying the foundation for a lifetime of mental well-being.

Brain-Boosting Foods & Nutrients for Different Ages

Understanding the nutritional needs of growing brains is critical for anyone involved in the upbringing of children. A child's brain undergoes a remarkable journey of growth and development from the time they are born all the way through adolescence. Just as crucial as ensuring they get enough sleep and exercise is recognizing the important role nutrition plays in brain development. The foods and nutrients we provide can significantly impact a child's cognitive abilities, emotional well-being, and overall development.

Infants and toddlers experience rapid brain development, and their dietary needs are uniquely tailored to support these changes. Nutrition in the first few years sets the foundation for lifelong brain health. During this time, essential fatty acids, particularly omega-3 fatty acids found in breast milk, formulas enriched with DHA, and oily fish like salmon, are fundamental. These fats build brain tissue and are critical for the development of visual and cognitive functions. Breastfeeding, where possible, is often recommended due to its comprehensive nutritional profile, including vital brain-boosting compounds (Innis & Elias, 2003).

As children transition into preschool and early school ages, their brains continue to seek nutrients, often reflected in their dynamic eating habits. Iron, necessary for transporting oxygen in the bloodstream, becomes vital. It's found in lean meats, beans, and fortified cereals. Iron deficiency during peak periods of growth can impair cognitive and psychomotor development in children (Beard, 2008). Incorporating a range of colorful fruits and vegetables provides antioxidants that protect the brain tissue from oxidative stress and enhances cognitive performance.

Once children reach school age, they begin to experience more consistent cognitive demands from learning environments, requiring a well-rounded nutritional strategy. Protein, crucial for neurotransmitter production, supports mental focus and cognitive processing. Offering lean meats, dairy, or plant-based sources ensures ample protein intake. Healthy carbohydrates in whole grains fuel the brain's energy needs and should be prioritized over simple sugars, which can lead to erratic energy levels and reduced concentration.

During adolescence, the brain undergoes another burst of growth, particularly in regions associated with decision-making and impulse control. Nutrition not only fuels this growth but aids in regulating mood and managing stress. B Vitamins, particularly B6, B9 (folic acid), and B12, are vital for nerve function and the synthesis of brain chemicals. Leafy greens, beans, and fortified foods are excellent sources. Given the increased autonomy of teens over their food choices, it's important to encourage healthy options that include these critical nutrients (Bryan et al., 2004).

Calcium and vitamin D, while traditionally associated with bone health, play significant roles in brain function as well. Calcium is involved in the release of neurotransmitters, while vitamin D receptors are present throughout the brain, indicating its contribution to cognitive health. Dairy products, fortified plant milks, and safe sun exposure can help meet these nutritional needs.

Let's not overlook the importance of hydration, often an underemphasized aspect of nutrition. Water facilitates mental clarity and cognitive processing, while even mild dehydration can impact attention and short-term memory performance in both children and teenagers. Encouraging regular water consumption instead of sugary drinks can have profound benefits on cognitive performance (Benton & Burgess, 2009).

Snack choices also significantly impact cognitive health. Instead of processed snacks, choose options rich in nutrients such as nuts, seeds, and whole fruits. Nuts like walnuts and almonds offer healthy fats and magnesium, which are both beneficial for brain health. A simple swap from chips to trail mix can make a positive difference in a child's learning capacity and mood.

Parents, teachers, and caregivers should aim to create an environment where nutritious, brain-boosting foods are readily available and appealing. Children's preferences are often shaped by repeated exposure and role modeling, so involving them in meal planning and preparation can be a valuable strategy. Encouraging children to explore a variety of foods fosters lifelong healthy eating habits that support not only their physical development but their cognitive growth and emotional well-being.

A balanced diet not only supports growth but can be instrumental in preventing developmental challenges and managing existing conditions. While no single food is a magic bullet, understanding how specific nutrients contribute to brain health can empower us to make informed choices that benefit our children's cognitive development. As we advance through this book, this information will provide a base from which to explore further the practical continuation of tailoring nutrition to complement other aspects of children's lives, such as sleep and exercise, creating a truly holistic approach to nurturing the mind.

Smart Snacking: Healthy Options for School, Home, and On-the-Go

Navigating the world of children's snacks is akin to walking through a minefield filled with colorful packaging and sugar-laden promises. Yet, when it comes to nurturing a child's cognitive and emotional development, smart snacking surfaces as a vital line of defense against the detrimental effects of poor dietary choices. Snacks, often seen merely as fillers, have the potential to enhance cognitive function and emotional well-being profoundly—if chosen wisely.

What constitutes a smart snack? Simply put, it's a snack that provides essential nutrients without compromising taste or convenience. The goal is to offer foods that fuel the brain while supporting long-lasting energy and mood stability throughout the day. For instance, combining carbohydrates with protein or healthy fats offers a balanced energy source that can help maintain focus and prevent energy crashes, which are often linked with sugary snacks (Benton, 2006).

When preparing children for school, the ideal snack should be easy to pack, shelf-stable, and free from common allergens. A mix of nuts and seeds, if allergies aren't a concern, offers protein and essential fatty acids like omega-3s, known to support cognitive health. Pairing these with dried fruits, rich in fiber and vitamins, or whole-grain crackers can create a well-rounded snack pack (Gómez-Pinilla, 2008). Safe alternatives might include sunflower or pumpkin seeds, offering the same punching dose of nutrients without allergenic risks.

Home snacking allows for more versatility and creativity. Kids can be involved in the preparation process, which not only helps them learn the importance of nutrition but also encourages them to try new foods. Some simple yet effective concoctions include yogurt parfaits layered with berries and a sprinkle of granola, or a classic combo of apple slices with almond or peanut butter. Both options provide vitamins, fiber, and healthy fats, fostering a nourishing environment for the brain and body (Bryan et al., 2004).

On-the-go situations often necessitate snacks that are portable and don't require refrigeration. Here lies the opportunity to use foods like whole-grain banana muffins, trail mix sans chocolate, or fresh fruits like bananas and clementines. These options hold up well to traveling and provide a complex mix of carbohydrates and fibers, preventing hunger-induced outbursts and maintaining concentration (Bellisle, 2004).

While cheese sticks and yogurt tubes serve as great dairy alternatives, always check labels for sugar content. Some brands sneak in excess sweeteners under the guise of fruit flavors. Speaking of sweetness, when a treat does fit the bill, aim for those made with natural sweeteners like honey or maple syrup, as opposed to high fructose corn syrup or artificial alternatives.

Liquids shouldn't be overlooked in any snacking scenario. Hydration, although often underrated, plays a fundamental role in cognitive performance. Consuming enough water can enhance memory functions and enhance mood stability in children (Popkin et al., 2010). Offering water infused with slices of citrus or berries introduces flavor without the drawbacks of sugary drinks.

Critically, it's about setting the right example and making snacking an intentional act rather than a mindless one. Teach children to view snacks as a means to nourish and energize their bodies, promoting better choices foundationally. In doing so, they learn to appreciate the balance and benefits of healthy snacking without the bondage of calorie counting or restrictive eating.

Teachers and caregivers can reinforce these practices in the school environment by advocating for policies that promote healthier snack options and by modeling conscious snack habits. Incorporating short lessons on nutrition into the school day can have long-lasting impacts, especially when children understand how their food relates to their capabilities and feelings.

In a world rife with convenience foods and fast-food options, the path to smart snacking for the mind can be paved with simplicity and clarity. Always remember: vibrant fresh foods, rich in color and texture, signal nutritional abundance. By refining snack choices, parents and caregivers fortify children's cognitive and emotional resilience and inspire positive lifestyle habits that might stand the test of time.

Ultimately, it's all about balance. Sure, there's place for occasional treats, but the core daily choices should be those that benefit the brain and body alike. With these mindful practices in play, smart snacking becomes an effortless way to complement the broader quest for a nourished, healthy mind.

Foods to Avoid: Processed, Sugary, and Harmful Additives

When supporting children's cognitive and emotional development, one can't ignore the impact of nutrition. While it's important to emphasize brain-boosting foods, it's equally critical to understand which foods could hinder progress. Processed foods, refined sugars, and harmful additives are often culprits that can interfere with healthy brain function.

Processed foods are ubiquitous in today's world, offering convenience at the expense of nutritional value. These foods are often high in unhealthy fats, refined sugars, and sodium, while lacking essential vitamins, minerals, and fiber (Monteiro et al., 2011). The refining process strips away the nutritional components that are vital for a child's brain development, leaving behind "empty calories" that contribute little more than energy without nourishing the body and mind. Foods such as instant noodles, packaged snacks, and ready-to-eat meals tend to fall into this category (Louzada et al., 2015).

The reasoning behind avoiding refined sugars goes beyond just physical health. Excess sugar consumption is linked to reduced cognitive function and emotional regulation in children (Khan et al., 2015). High sugar intake has been associated with attention deficits and hyperactivity, contributing to behavioral issues in some cases. Consuming sugary beverages, candies, and pastries can lead to energy spikes and crashes, impacting children's attention spans and moods. Limiting refined sugars can help maintain consistent energy levels and emotional stability, fostering a better environment for learning and development.

Artificial additives are another concern. These include preservatives, artificial colors, and flavor enhancers commonly found in processed foods. Some studies suggest a potential link between these additives and behavioral problems in children, including increased hyperactivity and difficulty concentrating (McCann et al., 2007). The body's response to these substances can vary, but minimizing exposure to artificial additives is a prudent step in promoting cognitive health.

Focusing on whole foods helps to counteract these negative influences. By choosing fresh fruits, vegetables, whole grains, and lean proteins, caregivers can ensure that children's diets are rich in nutrients needed for optimal brain function. Preparing meals from scratch may require more effort, but the benefits to a child's cognitive development and emotional well-being can be profound.

Beyond individual food choices, it is essential to consider the broader context of a child's eating patterns. Encouraging mindful eating habits, such as slowing down during meals and paying attention to hunger and fullness cues, can foster a healthier relationship with food. This not only aids in avoiding overeating but also helps in appreciating the natural flavors of whole foods, reducing reliance on processed options.

Education is equally important. Teaching children about the importance of nutrition and the effects of certain foods on their bodies can empower them to make informed decisions. When children understand the relationship between what they eat and how they feel or perform, they're more likely to choose foods that support rather than sabotage their growth.

It's also worth considering the environmental influences on diet. Children are often exposed to advertising for processed foods, which can shape their preferences and demands. Being critical of such media and providing age-appropriate guidance can help children become more discerning consumers. At the same time, involving children in meal planning and preparation can demystify healthy eating and make it an enjoyable part of their routine.

Reducing screen time during meals is another strategy that could enhance mindful eating practices. Mealtime offers an excellent opportunity for family connection and can be an arena for teaching valuable life skills, such as communication and patience—both of which are crucial for emotional and cognitive maturity.

In conclusion, avoiding processed foods, refined sugars, and harmful additives plays an essential role in supporting children's cognitive and emotional health. A diet focusing on whole, nutritious foods can significantly affect brain development, behavior, and emotional regulation. While convenience and marketing may push families towards less healthy options, informed choices and a proactive approach to nutrition can set children on a path of lifelong wellness.

Constant vigilance and small changes in dietary habits can lead to substantial improvements in brain health, supporting children as they learn, grow, and thrive. By embracing the power of whole foods and minimizing exposure to harmful substances, caregivers and educators can help nurture the next generation's cognitive and emotional capabilities.

The Role of Hydration in Cognitive Performance

Hydration is more than just a necessity for survival; it's a vital component for optimal brain function. The human brain is composed of approximately 75% water, and even mild dehydration can affect cognitive performance, affecting areas such as memory, attention, and mood. For children, who are in a crucial stage of cognitive and emotional development, maintaining proper hydration is essential. Dehydration can result in fatigue, irritability, and difficulty concentrating, all of which can hinder a child's learning process and emotional well-being (Benton & Burgess, 2009).

Understanding how dehydration impacts cognitive function begins with examining its effects on energy levels and mood. Studies have shown that dehydration can cause a reduction in cognitive performance, affecting short-term memory and the ability to process information efficiently (Popkin et al., 2010). This phenomenon occurs because adequate hydration ensures that cellular activities within the brain, including the transmission of neural signals, function smoothly.

When these cellular processes slow down, children may find it harder to focus and learn new information, which can impact their overall academic performance.

Moreover, hydration is crucial for maintaining both physical and cognitive activities. During strenuous activities or on hot days, children might lose water rapidly through sweat, which can impair cognitive functions if not compensated for with adequate water intake. It's not just about replacing lost fluids; it's about ensuring that bodily systems function optimally so that stress and tiredness do not creep in and affect a child's mental acuity (Adan, 2012). Parents, teachers, and caregivers play a vital role in encouraging kids to recognize their body's signals of thirst and respond appropriately.

In schools, providing easy access to water canisters or incorporating water breaks into the daily routine can significantly impact students' cognitive performance. Encouraging children to carry their own water bottles can also help, as it makes them more conscious of their hydration habits. Simply having a water bottle by their side can serve as a gentle reminder to stay hydrated throughout the day.

The challenges of maintaining adequate hydration are not limited to environmental conditions like heat and humidity. Sometimes, children's reluctance to drink water stems from preference, where flavored drinks or juices, also laden with sugar, become more appealing choices. Teachers and caregivers can creatively address this by infusing water with fruits like lemon or berries to make it more appealing without adding sugar, thus balancing hydration with nutritional health.

Educating children about the importance of hydration can be a powerful tool. Simple explanations about how water helps their brain function better can motivate them to drink more water. Including hydration as a part of health education classes could also emphasize its relevance, underscoring how drinking water is not only good for their growing bodies but also for their alertness and concentration during academic tasks.

The interconnectedness of hydration with other lifestyle factors should not be overlooked. A child's diet significantly influences hydration levels; meals rich in water content, such as fruits and vegetables, naturally contribute to a child's daily water intake. This not only helps in maintaining hydration but also ensures that other nutrients vital for cognitive functioning are consumed. Encouraging a diet that includes foods like watermelon, oranges, and cucumbers can be both an enjoyable and effective way to support hydration needs (Maughan, 2003).

Monitoring urine color can serve as an immediate and straightforward indicator of hydration status. Pale yellow urine is usually a sign of good hydration, while darker colors may suggest a need for more fluids. Encouraging children to be mindful of these signs can foster self-awareness, helping them manage their hydration proactively.

It must be noted, however, that overhydration, although rare, can also pose health risks, such as hyponatremia, where the body's electrolyte balance gets disrupted. This highlights the importance of teaching children to balance their water intake to meet their hydration needs without overconsumption. In this way, children learn to listen to their bodies, recognizing when they are thirsty without succumbing to the impulse to drink excessively.

In conclusion, hydration plays a pivotal role in supporting cognitive function in children. By fostering environments that promote adequate water intake and educating children about the benefits of staying hydrated, parents, teachers, and caregivers can positively influence their cognitive and emotional development. As we nurture the minds of the next generation, understanding simple yet profound influences like hydration will empower us to support children's learning and emotional well-being effectively.

Chapter 5: Sleep and Its Impact on Cognitive and Emotional Health

Sleep is not merely a nightly pause but a critical pillar that supports the cognitive and emotional scaffolding of a child's development. A well-rested brain is primed for absorbing new information and regulating emotions effectively, functioning akin to a fertile garden waiting to be sown with seeds of knowledge and resilience. When children receive adequate sleep, their brains consolidate memory and enhance learning abilities, leading to improved academic performance and better emotional regulation (Owens et al., 2016). Unfortunately, in today's fast-paced world, factors like screen time before bed, caffeine consumption, and even stress can disrupt the natural sleep cycles, consequently hampering the cognitive functions and emotional sensitivities that are crucial during formative years. Establishing consistent bedtime routines not only nurtures healthy sleep patterns but fosters an environment where a child's mind can flourish, creating a symbiotic relationship between rest and development. By understanding the science of sleep, parents and caregivers can make informed, empathetic decisions that prioritize and respect this essential component of holistic growth (Mindell & Meltzer, 2008).

How Sleep Supports Memory, Learning, and Emotional Regulation

Sleep isn't just a time of rest; it's a crucial part of a child's cognitive and emotional development. As parents, teachers, and caregivers, understanding the multifaceted role sleep plays in a child's well-being can empower us to foster environments that promote healthy sleep patterns. Let's dive into how sleep helps enhance memory, facilitates learning, and supports emotional regulation.

Firstly, when it comes to memory, sleep serves as the brain's personal organizer, helping to consolidate information acquired during the day. During different sleep stages, especially rapid eye movement (REM) sleep, the brain processes short-term memories and transfers them to long-term storage. This process is akin to a computer transferring files from volatile memory to a more permanent storage disk, ensuring that important data isn't lost. Interestingly, research has shown that sleep can influence both declarative (the facts and events) and procedural (the skills) memory, making it essential for both book learning and skill acquisition (Diekelmann & Born, 2010).

The link between sleep and learning is just as compelling. Children are constantly absorbing new information, and sleep plays a critical role in the retention and understanding of this knowledge. During sleep, particularly during stages where brain waves slow down, the brain reviews the experiences of the day, linking new material with prior knowledge. This integration helps children make sense of the world around them, promotes better comprehension, and boosts creativity. As a result, a well-rested child is more adept at tackling complex tasks and solving problems effectively the following day (Walker & Stickgold, 2016).

Beyond the cognitive benefits, sleep significantly impacts emotional regulation. A child who has sufficient rest is better equipped to handle stress and manage emotions. Sleep deprivation, on the other hand, can lead to irritable moods, heightened emotional sensitivity, and difficulty in managing behavior. This is because sleep affects the amygdala—the emotional center of the brain—and its interaction with the prefrontal cortex, which is responsible for executive function and impulse control

(Goldstein & Walker, 2014). Children who regularly miss out on sleep may face challenges in regulating their emotions, leading to behavioral issues both at school and at home.

Moreover, the relationship between sleep and emotional well-being is reciprocal. Not only does good sleep foster emotional health, but emotional distress can also disrupt sleep patterns, creating a challenging cycle that can be difficult to break. By establishing a consistent sleep routine and creating a soothing sleep environment, caregivers can help mitigate stressors that interfere with sleep, effectively supporting a child's emotional resilience (Gregory & Sadeh, 2012).

It's important for adults to recognize the diverse factors that might impact a child's sleep quality. Creating a supportive sleep environment involves more than ensuring a comfortable bed—it's about setting a bedtime routine that signals the body to wind down. This routine should ideally be free from stimulating activities, particularly screen-based ones, which can interfere with the body's natural sleep-wake cycle. Encouraging relaxing activities such as reading, listening to calming music, or doing simple mindfulness exercises can help signal to a child that it's time for rest.

Understanding the unique sleep needs at various developmental stages is essential too. Younger children and adolescents might have different sleep requirements, with rapid changes occurring in the structure and patterns of sleep during the transition to adolescence. These changes can often be accompanied by shifts in circadian rhythms, making it harder for teenagers to fall asleep early or wake up in time for school (Crowley et al., 2007). Recognizing and accommodating these changes can significantly impact their overall academic performance and emotional stability.

In essence, promoting optimal sleep isn't just about avoiding a cranky morning; it's a foundational piece in supporting a child's holistic development. As we consider the myriad ways sleep underpins memory retention, learning capacity, and emotional health, it becomes clear that it's not merely a passive state but an active partner in nurturing a child's potential. By prioritizing and modeling healthy sleep habits, we set children up for success in every aspect of their young lives.

Sleep Recommendations by Age Group

Sleep is a fundamental component of children's cognitive and emotional development, directly influencing their ability to learn, regulate emotions, and thrive in various environments. It's as vital as nutrition and exercise, and understanding how sleep needs change with age can help parents, teachers, and caregivers to provide the most supportive environment for growth and development. Let's dive into the specific sleep recommendations for different age groups, considering their unique physiological and psychological needs.

For infants, sleep is a cornerstone of brain development. Infants typically need around 14 to 17 hours of sleep per day, distributed across several naps and an extended night sleep. During these formative months, the brain is bustling with activity, consolidating learned experiences and establishing foundational neural connections (Hirshkowitz et al., 2015). Parents should encourage consistency by establishing a bedtime routine even at this early stage. Simple practices like a warm bath, gentle rocking, or a lullaby can signal to the infant's brain that it's time to wind down. Ensuring an environment that's conducive to sleep, such as a darkened room and a comfortable crib, further supports restful slumber.

Toddlers, on the other hand, require slightly less sleep, although it remains crucial. They need about 11 to 14 hours of sleep daily, including naps (Paruthi et al., 2016). At this age, establishing a consistent sleep schedule becomes essential as it fosters a sense of security and expectation. Predictability in routine helps toddlers transition from busy waking hours to winding down for the night. It's vital to limit stimulating activities and screen exposure close to bedtime as these elements can interfere with their ability to settle and interfere with the quality of sleep.

As children transition to preschool age, their sleep requirement drops to 10 to 13 hours a day. While naps are still common, they often start to phase out as children near school age. Night terrors and sleepwalking might appear during this stage and can disrupt sleep. However, most children naturally outgrow these issues. Maintaining a sleep environment that's safe and calm will help keep sleep disruptions to a minimum (Owens et al., 2014). Mindfully reading a story or practicing quieting down activities can also be beneficial pre-sleep rituals.

During the elementary school years, sleep needs decrease slightly. Children aged 6 through 13 need about 9 to 11 hours of sleep, which is a period of significant growth and learning. This is the age where social pressures begin to mount, and homework becomes a frequent evening activity. Balancing these demands with adequate rest can be challenging. Encouragement towards a consistent bedtime, avoiding caffeine, and creating a quiet time before bed are practical measures that foster quality sleep. Academics, sports, and social activities can quickly fill up after-school schedules, so it might be helpful to prioritize winding down at the end of the day to ensure children can manage stress and stay focused during school hours.

Adolescents, from ages 14 to 17, have unique sleep needs during a pivotal time of both physical change and social development. The recommended sleep duration is about 8 to 10 hours, but lifestyle choices and biological shifts often lead to insufficient sleep in this age group. The tendency to stay up late combined with early school start times often results in a chronic sleep deficit (Crowley et al., 2018). Educators and caregivers can encourage teens to optimize their sleep patterns by facilitating environments that align more closely with their developmental needs, such as advocating for later school start times or ensuring that teens understand the detrimental effects of blue light exposure and electronics before bed.

The role of sleep in learning and emotional regulation cannot be overstated. The REM (Rapid Eye Movement) sleep cycle, reaching its peak length later in the night, is particularly vital for regulating mood and storing memories. Thus, ensuring children and teenagers get enough continuous sleep is crucial for their emotional health and cognitive performance (Carskadon et al., 1993). While each child may have individual needs or variations, aligning sleep schedules with their natural rhythms helps maintain a healthy balance of sleep stages.

Understanding and applying these age-appropriate sleep recommendations can notably enhance a child's ability to manage stress, improve academic performance, and build a resilient emotional framework. It's a collaborative effort that involves creating consistent routines and an environment that responds to each child's evolving sleep needs. Ultimately, facilitating better sleep is about supporting long-term well-being, providing every opportunity for children to explore, learn, and develop in the healthiest way possible.

Sleep Disruptors: Late-Night Screens, Caffeine, Stress, and Overstimulation

Sleep is the cornerstone of cognitive and emotional health, especially for developing children. Despite its importance, various modern lifestyle habits can disrupt sleep patterns, leading to significant impacts on a child's brain development. Addressing these "sleep disruptors" is essential for parents, teachers, and caregivers who strive to nurture a healthy environment for children. This section focuses on four main disruptors: late-night screens, caffeine, stress, and overstimulation, and offers insights into how each can affect sleep quality.

In today's digital age, screens are ubiquitous—they're in homes, schools, and even cars. The blue light emitted by screens can interfere with the natural sleep-wake cycle, or circadian rhythm, by suppressing the production of melatonin, a hormone that promotes sleepiness (Cajochen et al., 2011). When children use devices close to bedtime, their brains are tricked into thinking it's still daylight, making it harder to fall asleep. Moreover, the stimulating content of many games and videos can further delay a child's bedtime. Reducing screen time in the evening and encouraging activities like reading can help mitigate these effects.

The widespread consumption of caffeine is another sleep disruptor that often goes unnoticed. While adults may reach for a cup of coffee, children are more likely to consume caffeine through a surprising variety of sources, including sodas, energy drinks, and even chocolate. Caffeine is a stimulant that blocks adenosine, the chemical responsible for sleepiness (Roehrs & Roth, 2008). Even moderate consumption can significantly delay sleep onset and decrease total sleep time in children. Parents should be mindful of what their children consume and consider alternatives to caffeinated beverages, especially in the afternoon and evening.

Stress is an inevitable part of life but becomes a concern when it leads to chronic sleep disruptions. School pressures, social dynamics, and even overly packed schedules can contribute to heightened stress levels in children. Stress triggers the release of cortisol, another hormone that can interfere with sleep (Pruessner et al., 1999). Teaching children stress management techniques, such as mindfulness and breathing exercises, can empower them to better manage their stress, promoting healthier sleep habits.

Overstimulation, both mental and physical, can also hinder a child's ability to wind down and drift into sleep. This often stems from a day packed with activities without any quiet time for relaxation. Constant engagement in high-energy activities or exposure to stimulating content can keep a child's mind and body in an alert state, unsuited for sleep. Creating a calming nighttime routine, where quiet activities replace stimulating ones, can help signal to the brain that it's time to prepare for rest.

Understanding and addressing these disruptors is crucial because sleep plays a vital role in a child's cognitive abilities and emotional health. During sleep, the brain consolidates memories, processes emotions, and clears out toxins that accumulate throughout the day. Insufficient or poor-quality sleep can impair attention, learning, and emotional regulation. Children become more likely to experience difficulties in school and social interactions, ultimately affecting their mental well-being (Mindell & Owens, 2010).

For proactive caregivers, it is essential to set up a supportive sleep environment and routine. Establishing consistent bedtime routines and environments can help children associate these cues with sleep time. Lowering lights, limiting noise, and ensuring a comfortable room temperature all contribute to a restful environment. Encouraging regular sleep and wake times can help regulate the circadian rhythm, promoting more consistent and restorative sleep.

In conclusion, the fight for healthy sleep among children is one worth undertaking, as it forms the backbone for both cognitive growth and emotional health. By identifying and mitigating disruptors like screens, caffeine, stress, and overstimulation, caregivers can empower children to nature positive sleep habits. In turn, this will provide a strong foundation for lifelong learning and emotional resilience.

Establishing a Healthy Bedtime Routine

Creating a consistent and healthy bedtime routine is vital for nurturing the cognitive and emotional well-being of children. It's particularly crucial because sleep has a profound impact on their ability to learn, remember, and regulate emotions. Recent studies highlight the crucial link between regular sleep patterns and improved academic performance and emotional resilience in children (Mindell et al., 2015). As such, establishing a healthy bedtime routine isn't just about getting kids to bed—it's about setting them up for success both in school and in life.

The journey to a good night's sleep begins long before the lights are turned out. It involves establishing a calming pre-sleep routine that signals to the brain and body that it's time to wind down. Ideally, this routine should start around the same time every night to help set the child's internal clock. Activities during this time might include taking a warm bath, reading a short story, or engaging in light stretches or calm breathing exercises. These activities can help lower cortisol levels and facilitate the production of melatonin, the hormone that promotes sleep (Gradisar et al., 2011).

One critical aspect of a bedtime routine is the environment in which children sleep. Their bedroom should be a sanctuary of calm—quiet, dimly lit, and free from distractions. Blackout curtains, white noise machines, and removing electronic devices from the room can significantly enhance the sleep environment. Studies have shown that minimizing light exposure and removing screens from the bedroom can improve both the duration and quality of sleep in children (Cain & Gradisar, 2010).

A nutritious snack that promotes sleep can also be part of the bedtime routine. Foods rich in tryptophan, an amino acid that the body converts into serotonin and melatonin, can facilitate sleep. Warm milk, turkey slices, or a small banana are excellent choices. However, it's essential to avoid caffeine and sugar-laden snacks before bed as they can interfere with sleep onset and quality.

Importantly, maintaining the same bedtime and wake-up time every day—even on weekends—fortifies a child's sleep schedule. While it might be tempting to let children stay up late or sleep in, particularly as a reward or during holidays, this can disrupt their sleep architecture and lead to issues like social jet lag, where their circadian rhythm gets out of sync (Wittmann et al., 2006).

Parents and caregivers can play a pivotal role in establishing and maintaining a consistent bedtime routine by modeling good sleep hygiene themselves. This includes setting aside time to wind down in the evening, aligning their sleep schedule with their child's, and being mindful of screen time in the hours leading up to bedtime. By doing so, adults not only support their sleep health but also set an example of prioritizing rest and relaxation.

An often overlooked component of bedtime routines is the importance of emotional check-ins before sleep. Spending a few minutes talking with children about their day—what went well, what they learned, and any worries they may have—can help alleviate stress and anxiety that might otherwise disrupt their sleep. This practice not only fosters a deeper connection between children and caregivers but also encourages the development of emotional intelligence.

Consistency in routines breeds security and structure for children. The predictability of knowing that sleep follows their nighttime ritual helps children relax and lowers resistance to going to bed. Structured routines can also help mitigate bedtime struggles, making it easier for children to fall asleep independently as they grow (Mindell et al., 2015).

In conclusion, establishing a healthy bedtime routine is a multi-faceted endeavor that requires thoughtful planning and consistency. By creating an environment conducive to sleep, incorporating calming activities, focusing on nutritional support, and maintaining regular sleep schedules, parents and caregivers can significantly impact their children's cognitive and emotional health. This foundation of good sleep practices will not only support brain development and emotional resilience today but instill habits that will benefit children into adulthood.

Chapter 6: The Power of Movement and Exercise

Movement and exercise are not just vital for maintaining physical health; they're also crucial for boosting cognitive function and emotional well-being in children. Regular physical activity enhances brain function by increasing blood flow to the brain, thereby fostering the growth of new neural connections and improving memory and learning capabilities (Hillman et al., 2008). Exercise also helps regulate emotions and reduce symptoms of anxiety and depression by triggering the release of endorphins, the body's natural mood elevators (Salmon, 2001). Encouraging kids to engage in a mix of aerobic, strength-building, and mind-body exercises can significantly benefit their focus and emotional regulation, particularly for those experiencing ADHD and related challenges (Pontifcx et al., 2013). By promoting active play and outdoor activities, parents and educators can support not only the physical but also the mental growth of children, setting a foundation for lifelong health and well-being.

Physical Activity and Its Connection to Brain Function

When we think about enhancing children's cognitive functions and emotional well-being, physical activity often takes a backseat to more direct interventions like academic tutoring or cognitive games. Yet, the link between movement and brain health is profound, deeply rooted in our biology and evolution. Physical activity doesn't just strengthen muscles – it supercharges the brain. We can better understand this connection by diving into scientific evidence and considering practical applications for children at various developmental stages.

In recent decades, researchers have uncovered the myriad ways in which physical activity benefits the brain. Regular exercise has been shown to stimulate the release of neurotrophic factors, which are proteins that aid in the growth, maintenance, and survival of neurons (Cotman & Berchtold, 2002). These factors enhance synaptic plasticity – the brain's ability to form new connections and strengthen existing ones. This plasticity is crucial for learning and memory, tying physical activity directly to cognitive functions critical for school performance and life skills.

Moreover, the prefrontal cortex, which governs executive functions like decision-making, problem-solving, and impulse control, benefits immensely from consistent physical activity. Studies indicate that children who engage in regular aerobic exercise show improved executive functioning levels compared to their less active peers (Hillman et al., 2014). This is particularly compelling for children struggling with attention-deficit/hyperactivity disorder (ADHD) or those who face difficulties in traditional learning environments. By incorporating regular movement into their routines, these children can experience better focus, enhanced mood, and greater academic success.

Yet the benefits of physical activity extend beyond improving cognitive functions. Physical exercise is a crucial component of emotional regulation in children. Activity causes the release of endorphins and serotonin, chemicals in the brain that act as natural mood lifters, reducing anxiety, depression, and other mood disorders (Dishman et al., 2006). Through regular movement, children can build resilience against stress, enhance self-esteem, and interact more positively in social settings. This emotional uplift not only bodes well for children's internal worlds but also for their interactions with peers and adults.

An essential consideration for parents, teachers, and caregivers is recognizing the diversity of physical activity options available. While structured sports can significantly benefit older children and teenagers, they aren't the only avenue. Yoga and mindfulness-based movement activities cater to both the body and mind, encouraging concentration and reducing stress. For younger children, active playtime involving running, jumping, and climbing offers a wealth of cognitive and emotional benefits. Such activities promote the development of motor skills, coordination, and balance, laying a critical foundation for complex cognitive tasks.

Importantly, physical activity interventions should not be one-size-fits-all. Each child's interests, developmental stage, and physical abilities must be considered to create an effective and enjoyable physical routine. Encouraging children to engage in physical activities they find enjoyable increases the likelihood of these habits persisting into adulthood – a vital consideration given the correlations between adolescent physical activity and adult health outcomes.

In today's digital age, where screen time often occupies much of children's free time, integrating movement into daily routines is more critical than ever. Simple strategies such as walking or biking to school, taking breaks for physical activities during long periods of study or screen time, and participation in family fitness activities can make a significant difference. As caregivers implement these small changes, they encourage a lifestyle where movement becomes a valued and integral part of children's everyday lives.

To achieve these goals, schools and communities can play a supportive role by creating environments that prioritize physical activity. By ensuring a minimum amount of daily physical education and promoting extracurricular physical activity programs, schools can be key partners in supporting children's brain health. Community parks and recreational facilities can also provide safe spaces for children and families to stay active.

In summary, the compelling evidence linking physical activity with improved brain function and emotional well-being makes a clear case for its prioritization in everyday life for children. By actively promoting varying forms of exercise that align with individual interests and capabilities, adults can cultivate a nurturing environment conducive to developing healthy brain architecture and emotional resilience. These investments in childhood movement today form the bedrock of a lifetime of cognitive and emotional strength.

Best Types of Exercises for Cognitive Benefits (Aerobic, Strength, Mind-Body)

When we think about exercise, the image of toned muscles and physical endurance often comes to mind. However, what's less visible but equally vital is the profound impact physical activity can have on the brain. For children, engaging in regular exercise doesn't just promote physical growth; it plays a critical role in cognitive development and emotional well-being as well.

Aerobic exercise, often referred to as cardiovascular activity, is an excellent starting point when considering activities that boost brain function. This type of exercise includes activities like running, swimming, and cycling. But why is it so effective for cognitive benefits? Aerobic exercises increase heart rate and improve blood circulation, delivering more oxygen and nutrients to the brain. This process not only supports existing neural connections but also fosters the growth of new ones. Research even suggests that regular aerobic exercise enhances memory and executive function in children, providing a solid foundation for academic achievement (Hillman et al., 2008).

Moreover, strength training has garnered attention for its cognitive benefits, particularly in older children and adolescents. While traditionally associated with building muscle, activities such as resistance exercises and weight training have been linked to improvements in working memory and concentration. Studies indicate that the increased neuromuscular demands during strength exercises can translate to enhanced neural efficiency and cognitive flexibility (Best, 2010). Schools and community programs offering strength-training activities provide opportunities for kids to not only develop physical capacity but also sharpen their mental acuity.

Then there are mind-body exercises, a category that includes practices like yoga, tai chi, and Pilates. These exercises are particularly effective for enhancing emotional regulation and mindfulness in children. Mind-body exercises involve intentional movements with an emphasis on breathing and mental focus. For children, engaging in these activities can reduce stress and anxiety levels while improving attention and self-regulation skills. Mind-body practices help strengthen the brain by activating areas involved in cognitive control and emotional processing, making them especially beneficial for children struggling with attention deficit disorders or anxiety (Verburgh et al., 2014).

Aside from the standalone benefits of each exercise type, incorporating a variety of these activities into a child's routine can have a synergistic effect. Aerobic exercises can elevate mood and energy levels, which makes it easier for children to engage in mind-body activities requiring focus and calm. On the other hand, the strength and muscular coordination developed through resistance training can enhance performance in aerobic sports, offering a well-rounded set of skills and benefits.

Parents, educators, and caregivers play an essential role in integrating these activities into a child's life. Creating an environment where kids are encouraged to explore and participate in different forms of exercise can lead to lifelong habits that support both physical and mental health. Building circuits of active play that incorporate games and exercises from each category can be especially impactful. The idea is to weave exercise seamlessly into daily routines, whether through structured sports, dance sessions, or playful activities like tag or obstacle courses.

Moreover, while structured activities are beneficial, unsupervised play should not be underestimated. It's typically during free-play that children learn social cooperation, risk assessment, and planning, which are vital executive functions. Encouraging children to participate in a mix of organized sports and free play supports their capacity to switch between structured activities requiring focused attention to more open-ended activities encouraging creativity.

In conclusion, a balanced exercise routine that includes aerobic, strength, and mind-body activities offers a rich spectrum of cognitive benefits for children. It supports healthy brain development and equips them with the emotional and mental tools required to navigate an increasingly complex world. The beauty of this approach lies in its simplicity and accessibility: no elite sports programs or gym memberships are necessary. All it demands is curiosity, imagination, and a little bit of movement each day—simple ingredients for a lifetime of health and cognitive vitality.

As we approach the end of this section, it's crucial to remember that every child is unique, and so too should be their approach to physical activity. Encouraging them to explore and interact with various types of exercises ensures they not only build cognitive agility but also a personal sense of accomplishment and joy in movement. Together, these practices are potent tools that can empower children, allowing them to thrive both mentally and physically.

How Movement Helps ADHD, Focus Issues, and Emotional Regulation

Imagine a classroom bustling with energy, where young students are encouraged to jump, swing, and move freely. It might look unconventional, but this environment fosters not just physical strength but improved focus, emotional balance, and better control over symptoms related to Attention Deficit Hyperactivity Disorder (ADHD). Science backs up what many have observed anecdotally: integrating movement into the daily lives of children significantly aids those struggling with ADHD and similar focus issues (Gapin et al., 2011).

Children diagnosed with ADHD often face challenges related to attention, impulsivity, and hyperactivity. These challenges can make traditional classroom settings difficult. However, introducing regular physical activity can offer a much-needed release, helping to limit these symptoms. Research suggests that aerobic exercise, in particular, plays a critical role by improving attention and reducing impulsivity. Exercise facilitates the release of neurotransmitters like dopamine and norepinephrine, which are crucial in maintaining attention and promoting focus (Pontifex et al., 2013).

The value of movement for emotional regulation cannot be understated. Children who engage in regular physical activity show fewer signs of emotional distress, anxiety, and depression. As kids move, they not only gain physical benefits but also experience a boost in self-esteem. This elevation in mood is often attributed to the endorphins released during exercise, contributing to a sense of happiness and calm that counteracts feelings of frustration and agitation common in children with ADHD and focus issues (Biddle & Asare, 2011).

By incorporating movement into the daily routine, children learn to manage their emotional responses better. This ability is particularly beneficial in high-stress situations, such as taking a test or speaking in front of a group. Regular physical activity helps build resilience, providing kids with the tools to approach challenges more calmly and confidently.

Schools and educators are increasingly aware of these benefits and are now designing programs that integrate movement into the curriculum. Flexible seating arrangements, like exercise balls and standing desks, offer subtly different ways for children to adjust and fidget without causing disruptions. Further, short activity breaks between academic lessons can refresh the brain and improve concentration when children return to their seats (Mahar et al., 2006).

It's important to consider the type of exercise that might be most beneficial. While aerobic exercises have been highlighted for their cognitive benefits, strength training and mind-body exercises such as yoga also contribute significantly to improving focus and emotional balance. Yoga, in particular, teaches mindfulness and breathing techniques that are invaluable for children who struggle with staying calm and focused. Engaging in these activities can instill a sense of discipline and self-awareness that supports long-term emotional growth.

Parents, too, play a significant role in facilitating their children's movement habits. Encouraging outdoor play and setting aside time for family activities can serve as a foundation for a physically active lifestyle. Simple practices like walking or biking to school, participating in dance routines, or limiting sedentary activities are excellent ways of promoting regular movement and exercise in day-to-day life.

The benefits of these practices go beyond individual wellness. Movement and exercise create opportunities for social interaction, which are poignant avenues for emotional development. Children learn teamwork, communication, and empathy when engaging in group sports or physical activities, further enhancing their emotional intelligence.

While the transition to a more active lifestyle may not immediately solve every attention-related challenge, it provides essential support. As a holistic approach, combining movement with other supportive strategies like a balanced diet, adequate sleep, and limited screen time sets the stage for improved cognitive function and emotional regulation.

Integrating purposeful movement into children's routines stands as a powerful tool to help them navigate the complexities of modern life. By harnessing the natural connection between body and mind, caregivers and educators give children the invaluable skill of self-awareness and control, fostering healthier, clearer-thinking young minds.

Ultimately, the goal isn't just about managing symptoms—it's about equipping children with skills they can carry throughout their lives. Viewing exercise as a critical component of a child's routine, especially for those with ADHD and focus issues, will lay the groundwork for healthier cognitive and emotional habits.

Physical activity is more than just exercise—it's a bridge to enhanced learning, emotional stability, and a brighter future for children who face unique challenges. Through thoughtful integration, movement can unlock more than just physical potential—it can liberate the mind.

Encouraging Active Play and Outdoor Time for Younger Kids

Sometimes, the simplest joys in life involve running around outside with nothing but boundless energy and a wild imagination. For young children, active play and outdoor time aren't just fun—they're essential for healthy development. Playing outside offers physical, cognitive, and emotional benefits that contribute significantly to a child's growth. When kids engage in unstructured outdoor activities, they're not just moving their bodies; they're also engaging their brains in ways that are crucial for developing various skills.

The cognitive benefits of outdoor play are substantial. The complexity of a natural environment—from uneven terrain to ever-changing weather conditions—offers children numerous opportunities to hone problem-solving skills. When climbing a tree or navigating a playground, a child learns to assess risk and make decisions—skills that are critical for cognitive flexibility. Research has shown a link between physical activity and increased brain function, highlighting the idea that moving and thinking are intertwined processes. According to a study by Koutsandréou et al. (2016), children who engage in regular physical activity tend to perform better on tasks that require executive function.

It's not just about cognitive development; emotional well-being is also fostered through outdoor play. The natural world offers a setting that's free from the pressures of structured environments and digital distractions. Time spent in green spaces has been shown to decrease levels of stress and anxiety, even in young children (McCurdy et al., 2010). Outdoor play can also promote resilience. When a child falls and scrapes their knee but gets back up to continue playing, they are learning perseverance. Such experiences build a child's character, making them more adaptable to life's challenges.

Feeling competent in physical activities boosts self-esteem, too. As children master new skills, like riding a bike or successfully crossing the monkey bars, they gain confidence. This self-assurance can spill over into other areas of their lives, empowering them to approach new tasks with enthusiasm and tenacity. Encouraging children to engage in various physical activities exposes them to a mix of challenges, ensuring balanced development of both fine and gross motor skills.

Parents, teachers, and caregivers can play a pivotal role in fostering active play by creating opportunities for diverse and flexible play experiences. Setting up playdates that focus on group activities can promote not just physical well-being but also social skills. Through team games and cooperative play, children learn how to communicate, negotiate, and collaborate, laying the foundation for effective interpersonal relationships. The social aspect of active play can be as valuable as its physical benefits.

Creating an environment that encourages exploration and curiosity is crucial. This can be as simple as providing access to a safe outdoor space where kids feel free to experiment and take calculated risks. In many neighborhoods, parks, gardens, and open fields offer excellent venues for active play, enabling children to interact with both peers and their surroundings. When children have regular access to these spaces, they're more likely to engage in activities that enhance their physical fitness levels while also benefiting their mental and emotional health.

Structured activities have their place, but the value of unstructured play should not be underestimated. Free play time, where children decide what they want to do, encourages creativity and decision-making. When a child directs their play, they become the storyteller, creating their worlds full of possibilities. Such activities stimulate imagination, which is a cornerstone of problem-solving and critical thinking. Children who spend ample time playing outdoors often exhibit higher levels of creativity and cognitive flexibility.

The role of schools is important, too. Incorporating outdoor physical education programs that emphasize both individual and team sports can foster a lifelong appreciation for physical activity. Moreover, schools can leverage nature's capacity to enhance learning by holding classes outdoors when weather permits. The benefits of being in nature don't stop with free play; they extend to structured educational activities, which can be more engaging and memorable when held outside the traditional classroom setting.

Lastly, adults must model active behaviors themselves. When children see their parents or teachers enjoying outdoor activities, they are more likely to want to participate as well. This shared time can enhance family bonds, offering adults the opportunity to impart values and life skills in an informal setting. Teaching children the joy of hiking, the peace of a quiet meadow, or the excitement of a community soccer game enriches their lives and lays a groundwork for a healthy, balanced lifestyle.

In conclusion, encouraging active play and outdoor time for kids may seem simple, but its impact is profound. By fostering environments that prioritize active play, we can support our children's physical health, cognitive development, and emotional well-being. In a world increasingly dominated by screens and structured schedules, the timeless experiences offered by outdoor play provide invaluable benefits that contribute to a happier and healthier childhood. Let's encourage our young ones to put down their devices, venture outside, and rediscover the world around them. Their bodies, minds, and hearts will thank us.

Best Brain-Boosting Exercises for Teens

As teenagers navigate the tumultuous years between childhood and adulthood, their brains are undergoing significant changes. The teenage brain is extraordinarily plastic, marked by a rapid development of neural pathways that support higher cognitive functions. In this sensitive period, engaging in appropriate physical exercises can offer substantial benefits not only for physical health but also for mental acuity, emotional regulation, and overall cognitive development. Let's explore some of the most effective brain-boosting exercises tailored for teens.

First and foremost, aerobic exercise stands out as one of the most impactful forms of physical activity for adolescent brain health. Activities such as running, swimming, cycling, or even a game of basketball can significantly boost heart rate, thereby increasing blood flow to the brain. This increase in cerebral blood flow nourishes brain cells and has been shown to enhance memory retention and concentration ("Hillman et al., 2008"). Scientifically speaking, regular aerobic exercise encourages the production of neurotrophins—proteins that support neuron survival and growth—which are critical for learning and memory.

Aerobic activities can also be a fantastic way for teenagers to release pent-up energy, helping them manage anxiety and stress more effectively. During these years, stress can often seem overwhelming, and having an outlet is crucial. It's important for caregivers to encourage teens to find an aerobic activity they genuinely enjoy, turning exercise into something they look forward to rather than another chore on their to-do list.

Strength training offers another avenue for brain enhancement, although it might not seem as obvious as aerobic exercise. Lifting weights or engaging in resistance exercises can improve mood and self-esteem ("Gordon et al., 2017"). These exercises often require a focus on form and precision, promoting mindfulness and concentration. More than just building muscle, strength training can help teens build discipline and resilience—skills that transfer to academic and social realms.

Another powerful tool in the exercise arsenal is mind-body exercises, with yoga and tai chi leading the pack. These disciplines teach mindfulness and balance, not only physically but mentally. The practice of yoga, for instance, has been associated with improved cognitive performance in adolescents. In a study on yoga's effect on teenagers, it was shown to enhance their executive functions, which include processes like planning, attention, and problem-solving ("Butzer et al., 2016"). By incorporating controlled breathing and focused movements, these practices help teens achieve a state of mental clarity and emotional calm.

Engaging in team sports also offers distinctive cognitive benefits due to the social component they inherently involve. Communicating with peers, strategizing in real-time, and fostering a sense of camaraderie can enhance a teen's social and emotional intelligence. Furthermore, these experiences often improve the ability to work effectively as part of a team and to handle both success and failure gracefully.

Exposing teenagers to varied types of movement, like dance or martial arts, could further enrich cognitive development. These activities demand coordination, which can improve the connections between the brain and the body. They also stimulate creativity and self-expression, allowing teens to explore their emotional landscapes in a safe, structured environment.

Incorporating brain-training exercises into day-to-day activities may also deliver cognitive gains. This could include activities that promote bilateral coordination—using both sides of the body synchronously. Exercises such as dribbling basketballs with both hands or practicing synchronized swimming engage different regions of the brain, enhancing connectivity and cognitive flexibility.

The timing and consistency of these physical activities are crucial. It's recommended that teens engage in at least 60 minutes of moderate to vigorous physical activity daily ("U.S. Department of Health and Human Services, 2018"). However, this doesn't have to be a continuous hour; it can be broken into smaller, manageable sessions throughout the day. The key is to establish regularity, making exercise a consistent part of their lifestyle, which can reinforce the creation of healthy habits that carry into adulthood.

Parents, teachers, and caregivers play an essential role in encouraging and facilitating exercise for teenagers. Providing opportunities and creating environments that make it easy for teens to engage in physical activities is paramount. This could involve enrolling them in sports teams, taking family bike rides, or simply encouraging active transportation like walking or biking to school.

It's also vital to focus on intrinsic motivation. Instead of emphasizing external benefits like weight control, the focus should be on the enjoyment and emotional benefits of physical activity. Helping teens find what they love—be it the sense of freedom in a morning run, the quietness of yoga, or the thrill of soccer—it facilitates a lifelong bond with exercise.

In conclusion, the teenage years are a critical period for developing cognitive abilities, emotional skills, and healthy habits. While the exercises and practices discussed here provide robust platforms for that development, they do more than just foster brain health. They help mold teenagers into well-rounded individuals prepared for the challenges of adulthood. By incorporating a variety of physical activities into their lives, teens can not only enhance their cognitive functions but also find balance, joy, and resilience.

Adopting these exercises can ensure that teens not only flourish academically but also thrive emotionally, offering them tools to navigate the complexities of growing up in a fast-paced world. As caregivers, the most valuable support we can provide is encouragement and understanding, facilitating an environment where physical movement is as vital and natural as anything else in their daily routine.

Chapter 7: Mental Stimulation & The Power of Reading

Mental stimulation plays a crucial role in children's cognitive and emotional development, and reading serves as a powerful tool in this process. Engaging with books not only nurtures intellectual growth but also fosters emotional intelligence, enhancing children's capacity to understand and navigate the complexities of human experiences. Reading trains the mind to concentrate, boosts memory retention, and sharpens comprehension skills, all of which translate into better academic performance and social interactions (Snow et al., 1998). The choice between physical books and digital screens can impact the reading experience, with studies suggesting that print books enhance comprehension and memory (Mangen et al., 2013). Additionally, immersing children in rich narratives, whether fiction or nonfiction, strengthens neural pathways and cultivates empathy and critical thinking (Nikolajeva, 2014). Encouraging diverse reading materials introduces children to new ideas and perspectives, broadening their knowledge base and teaching problem-solving in intricate scenarios. As parents, teachers, and caregivers, facilitating children's access to varied and appropriate reading material is invaluable in building their mental resilience and piquing their innate curiosity.

The Role of Reading in Cognitive Growth

Reading is a cornerstone of cognitive development, offering a profound impact that stretches across a child's entire lifetime. From the moment a child first engages with a book, a cascade of neural processes is initiated that supports brain development in various ways. Reading is not merely a skill to be acquired for academic success; it's a complex activity that enhances a wide range of cognitive abilities.

One of the most significant benefits of reading is its ability to enhance vocabulary and language skills. As children are exposed to new words and sentence structures, their linguistic abilities expand, enabling them to communicate more effectively and understand the world around them better. Research shows that the more children read, the more words they are exposed to, which is crucial during the sensitive periods of language acquisition (Mol & Bus, 2011).

Beyond vocabulary, reading stimulates greater cognitive engagement and critical thinking. Each story a child reads requires them to interpret meaning, predict outcomes, and draw inferences. This mental activity strengthens brain connectivity, particularly in areas responsible for language comprehension and emotional regulation. While processing the narrative, young readers often engage in mental visualization, fostering creativity and imagination. This imaginative play not only entertains but also allows children to explore hypothetical scenarios and develop problem-solving skills.

The act of reading itself encourages focus and attention, skills that are increasingly critical in our fast-paced, distraction-heavy world. When children read, they must concentrate on the text, follow its progression, and remember details from beginning to end. This process inherently improves memory retention and attention span. Studies have shown links between regular reading and improved cognitive abilities, including better memory recall and enhanced concentration levels (Wolf et al., 2016).

Social and emotional development is also closely tied to regular reading habits. Books often serve as mirrors and windows for young readers—mirrors reflecting their own lives and experiences, and windows offering glimpses into worlds they have yet to explore. This dual role helps foster empathy and social understanding as children gain insights into the thoughts, feelings, and perspectives of characters they encounter within stories (Mar et al., 2009). By learning to empathize with diverse characters, children develop a deeper understanding of human emotions and social interactions.

Additionally, the physical experience of reading can play a crucial part in cognitive development. While some may argue over the superiority of digital versus physical books, the tactile experience of holding a book, turning its pages, and scanning words line by line is believed to reinforce neural pathways related to comprehension and retention. Many educators suggest that physical books offer fewer distractions than digital screens, minimizing interruptions and encouraging sustained attention.

Despite these benefits, not all children find reading easy or enjoyable, especially in a digital age where screens compete for attention. That's why it's essential for caregivers and educators to create supportive environments that encourage reading as a pleasurable activity. Providing access to a variety of books—fiction and nonfiction alike—ensures that children can find subjects that genuinely interest them, fostering a lifelong love for reading.

In particular, reading fiction has been shown to improve empathy and emotional intelligence among children. When children immerse themselves in a fictional world, they practice stepping into characters' shoes, which teaches them to interpret and understand emotional cues. This kind of perspective-taking is invaluable, as it cultivates a sense of social awareness and an emotional repertoire that children can draw upon in real-world interactions.

In the context of non-fiction, books offer insights into factual data, processes, and phenomena that expand a child's knowledge base and cognitive frameworks. They teach critical thinking and analytical skills as children learn to sift through information, distinguish between fact and opinion, and apply knowledge in practical situations. By interacting with nonfiction, children develop the ability to understand complex topics, preparing them for higher academic challenges and everyday problem-solving.

A well-rounded reading diet contributes significantly to cognitive resilience and flexibility. Engaging with a range of genres and topics equips children with diverse experiences and knowledge, enhancing their ability to adapt to new situations and think creatively. This broad exposure boosts cognitive reserves, making it easier for them to connect seemingly disparate ideas and innovate solutions.

Encouragingly, promoting regular reading habits doesn't necessitate imposing intensive reading regimens. Instead, supporting choice, and nurturing curiosity can transform reading into a self-motivated desire. Creating habits such as reading out loud, setting aside dedicated reading times, and discussing books can integrate reading naturally into everyday life, providing consistent cognitive engagement.

Reading is not just a passive absorption of content, but an active dialogue between reader and text, fostering an interactive exchange that challenges and grows the mind. As caregivers, teachers, and parents, we must recognize our role in facilitating this interaction by providing access to engaging materials, modeling good reading behaviors, and supporting children as they navigate their literary journeys. Successfully embedding reading into the culture of childhood primes young minds for a lifetime of learning, adaptability, and empathy.

In summary, the value of reading in cognitive growth cannot be overestimated. It provides a critical foundation for linguistic, cognitive, social, and emotional development. By cultivating rich reading environments, we empower our children to thrive, not just in academic settings, but in every facet of their lives.

How Reading Enhances Memory, Attention, and Comprehension

Diving into the world of books doesn't just open up new horizons and adventures; it significantly augments a child's cognitive abilities, particularly in areas such as memory, attention, and comprehension. Let's explore how these three critical elements of cognitive development are influenced and enhanced by reading.

First and foremost, memory plays a crucial role in how children learn and retain information. Engaging with a well-written story requires the reader to remember details about characters, settings, plots, and subplots. This process naturally exercises their working memory—the ability to hold and manipulate information over short periods. According to research, the act of remembering and internalizing the sequences of a narrative can strengthen this cognitive function (Cain & Oakhill, 2007).

Reading also challenges long-term memory. When children recall facts and events from earlier chapters to make sense of new developments in a story, they're effectively training their brain to keep both short-term and long-term memories active, which can be beneficial in educational settings and everyday life (Pressley et al., 1998). Even more fascinating is how recognizing recurring themes and making predictions based on prior knowledge can enhance the ability to form lasting memories.

Attention is another pivotal skill that benefits from regular reading. The ability to focus on and absorb the content of a book often demands longer attention spans. In an age of constant digital distractions, reading requires young readers to tune out the noise and focus deeply on a single task. This depth of focus strengthens attention control—a useful skill when children need to concentrate during school or other demanding cognitive activities (Stevens et al., 2007).

Moreover, the narratives and content found in books can vary widely, from straightforward stories to complex texts that require critical thought. This variety plays a role in exposure to diverse vocabulary and concepts, thereby improving comprehension skills. Children who read widely have been found to develop better analytical skills, as they naturally learn to various interpret scenes, understand character motivations, and infer themes that aren't explicitly stated (Cain & Oakhill, 2007).

In many ways, reading offers a unique workout for the brain. When children encounter unfamiliar words, they learn to use context clues to deduce meanings, a process which enhances their inferential comprehension. By piecing together information, children aren't merely passive recipients; they become active participants in the discovery process, further building their cognitive toolkit.

The empathy aspect of reading can't be overlooked either. Literature, particularly fiction, places readers into the shoes of characters with different backgrounds and perspectives. Such exposure fosters emotional comprehension, allowing children to develop an understanding of feelings and motives. This is crucial for building not only cognitive but also social intelligence (Mar et al., 2006).

Finally, it's worth noting how reading reinforces brain plasticity. By consistently challenging and engaging the brain with new narratives and information, reading fosters neural connections that contribute to a child's mental flexibility and adaptability. This neuroplasticity ensures that as children grow and their brains evolve, they remain open to learning and adapting to new challenges, effectively setting the stage for lifelong cognitive health.

Fostering a love for reading in children can thus be one of the most effective ways to enhance their memory, attention, and comprehension. Creating a reading routine at home or in classrooms, surrounding children with a variety of books, and discussing stories can further encourage a culture of curiosity and lifelong learning. This habit not only equips children with the cognitive skills needed for academic success but also prepares them for the complexities of human relationships and emotional intelligence.

Ultimately, the role of reading in a child's development exemplifies the profound impact of seemingly simple activities. In supporting children on their journey through literature, we provide them with tools to navigate both their academic and personal worlds with greater confidence and understanding.

Physical Books vs. Digital Screens: Does It Make a Difference?

The question of whether physical books or digital screens are better for children's reading and cognitive development sparks lively debate. Parents, teachers, and caregivers often wonder which format provides more mental stimulation and fosters better learning outcomes. As technology advances rapidly, the need to understand the impact of these media on the mind becomes crucial, particularly for developing brains.

First, let's look at physical books. These traditional reading tools offer a sensory-rich experience due to their tactile nature, the smell of the paper, and even the sound of turning pages. Research shows that the tactile feedback from handling a book can improve memory retention (Mangen & Kuiken, 2014). Kids flipping through a book learn to associate the physical act with the storyline, building spatial and cognitive mapping skills that enhance comprehension. Moreover, seeing the visual progress—pages turned and chapters completed—often gives children a tangible sense of achievement, boosting their motivation to continue reading.

Beyond the tactile elements, reading physical books involves fewer distractions. Unlike digital devices, books don't come with notifications, pop-ups, or the temptation of multitasking. This uninterrupted focus helps children to immerse themselves fully in the story, promoting deep reading and better understanding (Wolf, 2018). Parents and teachers can also engage in more meaningful discussions about the content when children are not distracted by digital interruptions.

Now, consider digital screens. While critics often point out the downsides, they do offer some unique benefits. Digital platforms can provide interactive elements such as animations and hyperlinked content that engage children differently and might appeal to visual learners (Liu et al., 2016). E-books can be particularly useful for reluctant readers by including features like adjustable text size and built-in dictionaries. Furthermore, carrying an entire library on a single device encourages reading anywhere, anytime, potentially increasing the time kids spend with books.

However, digital reading comes with significant challenges, especially for younger children who need more guidance on self-regulation. The potential for distraction is much higher with digital devices. Children can quickly shift away from reading to gaming or social media, reducing their focus on the task at hand. Screen glare and blue light are other concerns, as they may lead to eye strain and disrupt sleep patterns if devices are used before bedtime.

In evaluating the impact of these formats on cognitive development, it's crucial to consider the context in which they are used. If digital screens are integrated thoughtfully, they can complement traditional reading and provide diverse educational opportunities. For instance, interactive e-books that include exercises or quizzes can reinforce what young readers learn, offering immediate feedback to strengthen understanding. Yet, moderation and a balanced approach are key to preventing the potential downsides.

Another factor to consider is the reading material itself. Whether on paper or a screen, the content's quality and complexity play pivotal roles in stimulating cognitive growth. Carefully chosen books, whether fiction or nonfiction, can enrich a child's vocabulary, enhance empathy, and broaden worldviews. It's the substance of what children are reading that might matter most, even more than the format.

So, is one format superior to the other? That largely depends on individual needs, preferences, and situational contexts. Some children and parents may prefer the ease and accessibility of digital screens, while others cherish the sensory richness of physical books. Blending both could be a feasible strategy, allowing kids to benefit from different aspects of each medium. By supplementing physical books with digital content, caregivers can cater to varying learning styles and situations.

To conclude, striking a balance between physical books and digital screens is likely the wisest choice, maximizing benefits from both. Encouraging children to enjoy reading in its many forms fosters not only cognitive benefits but also a lifelong love of learning. By understanding each medium's strengths and weaknesses, parents, teachers, and caregivers can make informed decisions that align with their child's developmental needs and optimize their reading experiences.

Why Reading Fiction & Nonfiction Both Strengthen Brain Pathways

Delving into the world of reading, we uncover an activity that's not just about turning pages and absorbing stories. Reading both fiction and nonfiction provides children with a dynamic mental workout, enhancing various cognitive skills and fostering neural development. From an early age, reading becomes a gateway to building stronger, more adaptable brain pathways. Exploring the distinct benefits of fiction and nonfiction offers valuable insights into how they collectively contribute to robust brain development.

Research indicates that fiction and nonfiction stimulate different cognitive processes, effectively complementing each other in strengthening brain pathways. Fiction engages areas of the brain associated with empathy and emotional intelligence. By immersing themselves in fictional worlds, children practice perspective-taking, understanding motivations, and predicting behaviors, which mirror real-life social situations. These activities activate the brain's default mode network, which is crucial for empathy and theory of mind development (Mar, 2018).

Meanwhile, nonfiction reading sharpens analytical and critical thinking skills. By interacting with factual content, children learn to process information systematically, evaluate evidence, and form logical conclusions. This genre of reading engages the brain's executive functions, which are responsible for decision-making, problem-solving, and controlling cognitive processes (Ngo, 2020). Nonfiction reading can cultivate an inquisitive mindset, motivating children to question the world around them and search for evidence-based answers.

The synergy between fiction and nonfiction provides a holistic cognitive workout. A balanced diet of both genres ensures that young minds can empathize and reason effectively. Moreover, children who exhibit a blend of empathy and analytical skills often excel not only academically but also in interpersonal scenarios. These skills are intertwined with executive functioning, providing children with the tools necessary for navigating complex social dynamics and academic challenges (Zunshine, 2021).

An intriguing aspect of combining fiction and nonfiction reading lies in their shared ability to enhance memory retention and comprehension. When narrative elements from fiction are combined with the factual knowledge of nonfiction, children create intricate mental maps that facilitate long-term retention. The storytelling nature of fiction, with its ordered sequence and emotional involvement, aids in encoding information in the brain's episodic memory, improving recall and comprehension (Brookshire, 2019).

Nonfiction equally contributes to this process by providing context and background information. By correlating engaging narratives with verified data, children develop a multifaceted understanding of topics. This not only enhances memory retention but also boosts vocabulary acquisition and linguistic skills, paving the way for improved academic performance and eloquence in expression.

But why is this important for cognitive development? The brain, a highly plastic organ, thrives on varied and enriched experiences. Neuroplasticity, the brain's ability to reorganize itself by forming new neural connections, is a vital mechanism in learning. Both fiction and nonfiction reading stimulate neuroplasticity, as they require active engagement, imagination, and reasoning (Kidd & Castano, 2013). This plasticity facilitates the development of stronger brain pathways, optimizing the brain's efficiency and adaptability.

Furthermore, reading diverse genres helps maintain cognitive flexibility—a crucial skill in life. Cognitive flexibility, or the ability to switch between thinking about different concepts, enables children to adapt to new environments, challenges, and perspectives. By exposing children to a variety of genres, we are essentially training their brains to be more adaptable and resilient in the face of novel situations (Gurman et al., 2015).

The benefits of reading fiction and nonfiction are not confined to cognitive gains alone; emotional development also reaps rewards. Fiction encourages children to explore emotions, sympathize with characters, and understand complex emotional landscapes. This enriches emotional intelligence, a key factor in forming healthy relationships and managing emotions effectively. Nonfiction, on the other hand, offers reality-based insights, grounding emotional understanding in factual experiences and real-world applications.

As parents, teachers, and caregivers, fostering a love for both fiction and nonfiction reading can seem like an overwhelming task. But it doesn't have to be. Simple strategies, like setting up a reading routine, offering a diverse selection of books, and engaging in discussions about what children read, can significantly enhance their reading experiences. It's essential to remember that the goal isn't just to read a certain number of books but to cultivate a lifelong love for reading that will fortify their cognitive and emotional development.

Finally, it's worth acknowledging the role of reading in today's digital age. While digital platforms provide access to an ever-expanding repository of information, they can't substitute the tactile and immersive experience of reading physical books. Encouraging children to read both fiction and nonfiction books in print can reduce distractions and foster deeper engagement. Print materials offer fewer interruptions, enabling children to develop sustained focus and comprehension skills, critical elements in optimizing brain development.

In conclusion, both fiction and nonfiction are invaluable resources in a child's cognitive and emotional development. Their unique and complementary strengths bolster brain pathways, fortifying a child's capacity to think critically, empathize, and adapt to life's myriad challenges. Whether navigating fantastical realms or exploring the intricacies of the real world, reading offers a foundation for lifelong learning and cognitive resilience. As we guide our children in their reading journeys, we're equipping them with tools not merely to understand the world but to transform it.

The Link Between Reading & Emotional Intelligence

Reading is often seen purely as a cognitive exercise, but its benefits extend well beyond. Emotional intelligence (EI) is intricately woven into this seemingly solitary activity, offering far-reaching advantages for a child's social and emotional growth. Understanding emotions, developing empathy, and improving interpersonal skills are just a few areas where reading profoundly impacts a child's emotional intelligence. Books become tools for readers to journey through complex emotional landscapes, allowing them to better understand their own feelings and those of others.

When children dive into a story, they don't just decode words and sentences; they engage in an emotional simulation. This engagement allows them to live vicariously through characters, experiencing a spectrum of emotions and situations. Such experiences are invaluable in developing empathy. Researchers have found that consistently reading fiction can improve one's ability to empathize with others. In fact, a study conducted by Kidd and Castano in 2013 found that reading literary fiction improves a reader's Theory of Mind, a crucial aspect of empathy that involves understanding others' thoughts and feelings (Kidd & Castano, 2013). By immersing themselves in diverse lives and perspectives, children gain tools to navigate their real-world social environments.

Consider how reading fiction offers children scenarios where they encounter moral dilemmas. As they analyze characters' motives and intentions, they exercise critical thinking and emotional evaluation. This process mirrors real-life interactions where assessing others' feelings and motivations is essential. Reading, in this way, becomes a mental rehearsal space where children practice these skills safely and creatively. Moreover, it introduces them to complex situations beyond their immediate experience, enhancing their ability to respond empathetically to others' needs and feelings in real life.

Interestingly, while fiction gains much recognition for boosting emotional intelligence, non-fiction shouldn't be underestimated. It offers significant value by providing insights into cultural, historical, and psychological contexts. Understanding these contexts enables children to relate better to people from diverse backgrounds, fostering emotional intelligence by appreciating differences and commonalities among humans. This is particularly important in today's increasingly globalized world, where cross-cultural understanding plays a pivotal role.

Engaging with books that explore emotional or psychological themes also contributes to building emotional intelligence. Titles that specifically address emotions, feelings, or interpersonal relationships can serve as guides for children to understand their emotional landscape. Such books might tackle themes like bullying, friendship, or family dynamics, prompting reflections on feelings and better emotional regulation. These reflections translate into improved emotional awareness, a cornerstone of emotional intelligence.

In addition to the emotional insights gleaned from reading, the environment surrounding the reading experience also matters. When adults participate in reading activities with children, they augment the process by discussing themes, characters, and emotions. Asking open-ended questions about a character's actions or feelings can facilitate critical dialogue and emotional discourse, reinforcing the connection between reading and emotional intelligence. This interaction rarely occurs in digital reading environments, highlighting the importance of physical books and the shared experiences they spark.

Moreover, discussing books with peers or in group settings provides children opportunities to express their interpretations and emotions openly. Book clubs or reading groups not only encourage reading habits but also enhance social bonds through shared experiences. Children learn to listen, express opinions, and engage in meaningful dialogues with peers, refining their communication skills and emotional intelligence through the richness of communal reading activities.

In the grand tapestry of cognitive development, the role of reading transcends mere knowledge acquisition. It fosters emotional growth and cultivates a deep understanding of self and others. The act of reading becomes a dynamic interplay of cognition and emotion, sculpting well-rounded individuals who can navigate the complexities of human interactions with empathy and insight.

Often, overlooked is the role of emotional intelligence in academic achievement. Children with higher emotional intelligence tend to perform better academically. They involve themselves more deeply in learning experiences due to their enhanced ability to manage stress, collaborate with peers, and maintain motivation. As they grow, these skills build resilience and adaptability, crucial traits for lifelong learning and personal growth.

In conclusion, as parents, caregivers, and educators, recognizing the profound impact of reading on emotional intelligence offers a powerful tool to nurture children's development. By incorporating diverse and emotionally challenging literature into children's routines, adults can lay the groundwork for more empathetic, socially adept, and emotionally intelligent individuals. The stories found in the pages of a book are not just words; they are gateways to a deeper understanding of the human condition, seamlessly blending cognitive and emotional realms for enriched personal growth.

Brain Training & Cognitive Exercises

In today's fast-paced, technology-driven world, nurturing a child's cognitive development through brain training and cognitive exercises is more crucial than ever. These exercises aren't just about enhancing academic performance; they're pivotal in building foundational skills that support emotional regulation, critical thinking, and problem-solving abilities. As children grow and face new challenges, providing them with the right cognitive tools can make a significant difference not only in their educational journey but also in their overall well-being.

From an early age, engaging children in activities that stimulate their brain can lay the groundwork for lifelong learning. Simple games like puzzles, memory challenges, or even strategic board games such as chess or checkers offer immense benefits. These activities encourage children to think critically, plan ahead, and develop strategies, which are essential skills in both academic and real-world settings (Gray, 2015). Such games help strengthen neural pathways and promote the development of executive functions, which oversee self-regulation, planning, and task flexibility (Diamond, 2013).

Cognitive exercises don't just benefit children academically; they also enhance social skills. Participatory games and activities teach children the importance of cooperation, communication, and empathy. When kids play together, they're not only learning to share and take turns but also developing the ability to see situations from others' perspectives. This kind of empathetic understanding is a vital component of emotional intelligence and social competence (Gopnik et al., 1999).

Beyond traditional games, introducing brain training through structured exercises can provide an additional layer of cognitive stimulation. Programs designed to improve memory, processing speed, and attention are becoming increasingly popular among parents and educators. While some skepticism surrounds the actual efficacy of such programs, studies have suggested that consistent and focused training can lead to moderate improvements in cognitive performance, especially when combined with other supportive activities (Melby-Lervåg & Hulme, 2013).

Incorporating technology into brain training isn't inherently negative, and when used judiciously, it can complement traditional learning methods. For instance, interactive apps that adapt to a child's performance can provide personalized learning experiences that challenge and motivate children to surpass previous limits. However, it's essential to ensure that screen time is balanced with other forms of active play and offline learning to avoid overstimulation (Munakata et al., 2004).

A crucial aspect of cognitive exercises is flexibility and variation. Just as muscles need different types of workouts to grow and strengthen, the brain benefits from diverse challenges. A blend of activities that require analytical thinking, creativity, and physical movement should be incorporated into a child's daily routine. Activities like solving math puzzles, engaging in storytelling or creative writing, and practicing musical instruments can significantly broaden a child's cognitive capacities (Habibi et al., 2016).

One often overlooked but highly effective cognitive exercise is teaching children mindfulness practices. Simple activities like guided meditation or focused breathing can help children develop better attention spans and emotional regulation skills. These practices foster an increased awareness of thoughts and feelings, which can contribute to better stress management and decision-making (Kalmanowitz et al., 2012).

Developing a consistent habit of reading is another potent cognitive exercise. Encouraging children to read a variety of genres fosters imagination and comprehension skills and provides an opportunity to learn new vocabulary and concepts. Reading fiction has been shown to improve empathy and social understanding, as it allows readers to experience diverse perspectives and emotions (Mar et al., 2006).

Parents, teachers, and caregivers play a pivotal role in facilitating cognitive exercises. By actively engaging in these activities alongside children, adults can provide guidance, encouragement, and a shared sense of achievement. This involvement not only strengthens the child's learning but also builds a supportive environment where mutual interest in cognitive growth is evident. By finding joyful and cooperative ways to participate in these exercises, the bond between caregiver and child can be strengthened, fostering an environment rich with support and understanding.

The journey of brain training and cognitive development is ongoing, and patience is paramount. Results are not immediate, and it's vital to appreciate the incremental progress and celebrate small achievements. What matters is consistency and the scaffolding of varied and enriching experiences that cumulatively build a resilient, adaptive, and well-rounded mind ready to embrace the world. Through these efforts, caregivers can empower children, helping them navigate life's complexities with confidence and competence.

Teaching Critical Thinking and Problem-Solving Through Reading

Reading is often celebrated for its ability to transport us to different worlds, but it's also a powerful tool for teaching critical thinking and problem-solving. When children engage with books, they are not just passively absorbing information; they are actively making connections, questioning narratives, and considering multiple perspectives. This dynamic process helps them develop key cognitive skills that are essential for navigating the complexities of real-world situations.

At its core, critical thinking involves analyzing information, evaluating evidence, and synthesizing insights to form a reasoned judgment. Reading, particularly when approached interactively, nurtures these abilities by requiring children to discern the motivations of characters, predict plot developments, and confront moral dilemmas. For example, when a child reads a mystery novel, they must piece together scattered clues to solve the story's puzzle, enhancing their ability to think logically and critically.

Books offer scenarios where the answers are not always black and white, and children are prompted to explore gray areas and ambiguities. This opens the door for discussions about right and wrong, fairness, and empathy—integral components of problem-solving. Literature like "To Kill a Mockingbird" or "The Giver" challenges readers to grapple with societal norms and morals, fostering a sense of empathy and ethical reasoning. Such experiences prepare children to address real-life problems with a balanced and well-informed mindset.

Moreover, reading diverse genres—from science fiction to historical accounts—stimulates a child's ability to envision numerous possibilities and outcomes. It encourages them to ask "what if" questions, a crucial practice in problem-solving. A study by Mar et al. (2006) suggests that exposure to fiction is associated with better social ability and a stronger understanding of complex social relationships, indicating that reading fiction may support the development of social and emotional intelligence, both vital for effective problem-solving.

Interactive reading sessions can further enhance these skills. When parents and teachers ask open-ended questions about a book's content, they invite children to express their interpretations and reasoning. Questions like "Why do you think the character made that choice?" or "What would you do differently?" help guide children in constructing their arguments and considering the motivations behind different decisions.

Incorporating discussions on the structure, language, and themes of a book can also help children understand the nuances of persuasive writing and rhetoric. By analyzing how authors balance varying viewpoints, children can learn to apply similar strategies in their thought processes and communications. This analytical practice aligns with Bloom's Taxonomy, which categorizes critical thinking, problem-solving, and analysis as higher-order skills (Krathwohl, 2002).

Recognizing patterns, an essential aspect of cognitive development, is another skill honed through reading. By identifying and understanding narrative patterns, children develop a greater ability to anticipate outcomes and devise solutions to new problems. A child who has explored the themes of transformation in books like "Alice's Adventures in Wonderland" can generalize that understanding to real-world scenarios, such as how changes in their environment might influence their own lives.

Besides individual growth, reading together fosters a shared learning experience that helps build collective problem-solving skills. Reading circles, book clubs, or family reading nights encourage children to articulate their thoughts and listen to others, developing communication skills critical for collaborative problem-solving. This social interaction also introduces the idea that problems can be solved collaboratively, leveraging the unique strengths and perspectives of a group.

Importantly, while digital platforms and interactive apps are popular today, they should complement, not replace, the tactile experience of reading physical books. Engaging with real, tangible texts demands focus and reduces the distractions commonly associated with screens, allowing deeper concentration and fostering a connection with the material (Mangen et al., 2013).

As educators and caregivers, creating an environment that treasures books and reading as tools for cognitive development can significantly impact a child's ability to navigate future challenges. Providing access to a wide range of reading materials, offering time for reflection, and encouraging discussion can cultivate a lifelong love of reading, equipping children with the critical thinking toolkit necessary for problem-solving.

Ultimately, reading is not just an activity; it's an invitation. An invitation to explore, question, and dream. It's a journey that shapes how children make sense of the world and their role within it. By prioritizing reading as a medium for teaching critical thinking and problem-solving, we empower our children to become thoughtful and capable stewards of their own futures.

The Benefits of Learning a Second Language or Musical Instrument

When we think about mental stimulation for children, the learning of a second language or the mastery of a musical instrument often surface as powerful avenues. These activities aren't just enriching; they're transformative in ways that are deeply rooted in brain science. Let's delve into how these skills provide mental workouts that can help develop the cognitive and emotional facets of a child's brain.

Mastering a second language involves a comprehensive engagement of the brain, compelling it to operate much like a mental gym. While navigating between two linguistic systems, the brain exerts multiple executive functions—those crucial processes like problem-solving, multitasking, and attention control. Bialystok et al. (2009) suggest that this complex juggling task enhances what psychologists term "cognitive flexibility." In practical terms, this ability allows children to switch gears more smoothly and adapt to new information—a skill that's beneficial far beyond the classroom.

Similarly, learning a musical instrument offers its own unique set of cognitive benefits. Research underscores the relationship between musical training and the enhancement of auditory processing abilities. Kaminski et al. (2017) assert that musical training changes brain structures involved in the processing of sound, improving the ear's ability to distinguish subtle differences in pitch and rhythm. This heightened auditory acuity can support language processing and literacy skills, creating better readers and communicators.

There's something inherently emotional about connecting with music. It reaches into the emotiònal centers of the brain, offering an expressive outlet that's particularly important for children navigating the complexities of growing up. Playing an instrument allows children to express themselves without words and to communicate emotions they might not yet fully understand. Music's role in emotional expression and regulation is well-documented, serving not just as a means of expression but also as a pathway to emotional health and resilience.

On a social level, involvement in musical activities or language learning frequently positions children in group settings—be it a band, choir, or language club—where teamwork and collaboration come into play. These environments can enhance social skills and build camaraderie. According to a study by Barrett (2014), shared musical experiences can foster a greater sense of belonging and social cohesion among young participants, supporting emotional and social well-being.

Additionally, the act of learning can fundamentally change how a young brain is wired through neuroplasticity, the brain's ability to reorganize itself by forming new neural connections. This adaptability is particularly pronounced in childhood, meaning that the benefits of learning languages or music can be profound and long-lasting. Enhanced memory, improved problem-solving skills, and refined auditory functions are just a few of the cognitive improvements that persist into adulthood, nurtured by the neuroplastic nature of a developing brain.

It's also worth noting the motivation and perseverance required to learn a language or instrument. These activities are not mastered overnight and require sustained effort and practice. Thus, they inadvertently teach children the value of grit and persistence. A child engaged in such learning endeavors often becomes more adept at managing setbacks and failures, viewing them as part of the learning process rather than insurmountable obstacles.

In incorporating these activities into a child's routine, the goal isn't just about adding another skill to their resume. It's about embedding practices that fundamentally enrich their cognitive toolkit and nurture their emotional resilience. Whether through the syncopated beats of a drum or the lilting tones of a new language, children are engaging in workouts for their most vital organ: the brain.

Indeed, the benefits of learning a second language or a musical instrument extend beyond individual cognitive skills; they weave into the fabric of a child's life, influencing how they think, feel, and interact with the world around them. By encouraging such endeavors, parents, teachers, and caregivers aren't just nurturing young musicians or bilingual speakers; they're cultivating thinkers, creators, and emotionally intelligent individuals ready to navigate the intricate dance of life's challenges and joys.

The Right Balance Between Structure and Free Play

Finding the sweet spot between structure and free play in children's reading habits can be pivotal for cognitive and emotional development. The challenge lies in structuring activities without stifling creativity or discouraging the natural curiosity that drives learning. When managed wisely, the balance between these two can stimulate a child's mind, develop critical thinking, and foster a lifelong love of reading.

Structuring reading time doesn't have to be rigid or overly prescriptive. In fact, creating a literacy-rich environment supplemented with books accessible just about anywhere in the home or classroom can accomplish wonders. This approach encourages children to be spontaneous about their interest in books, which can lead to unprompted reading sessions. The key is to guide them to explore a variety of genres and topics, which helps to build a broad and flexible cognitive framework that can support complex problem-solving in the future (Dweck, 2006).

On the other end of the spectrum, free play should explicitly include unstructured reading time, where children can choose whatever attracts their attention. Free play is crucial for fostering creativity. While they may initially gravitate toward material that seems trivial or less challenging, this autonomy often enhances intrinsic motivation. When children are motivated for the pleasure of discovery, their brains develop stronger connections, facilitating more effective learning and memory retention (Siegel, 2012).

Research supports the idea that balanced reading activities can stimulate different parts of the brain, thereby enhancing cognitive skills and emotional health. A study on reading interventions showed that when encouragement to explore was paired with moments of structured learning, children demonstrated improved reading comprehension and a more profound emotional understanding (Thomas & Johnson, 2019). Such an approach promotes using both logical and creative skills, setting the foundation for emotional intelligence.

Giving children choices in what they read while embedding structured activities like book discussions can present the best of both worlds. Discussions encourage children to articulate their thoughts and bolster comprehension while also teaching them valuable social and emotional skills, such as empathy and perspective-taking. The conversations that arise during these sessions can stretch their minds while promoting understanding of the material in a social context (Siegel, 2012).

It's also beneficial to associate reading with positive emotions. For instance, a cozy reading nook can be a simple yet effective way to foster a child's ability to focus and absorb content deeply. Similarly, family reading time can make the activity feel engaging and emotionally rewarding. When parents or caregivers participate in reading, they model focused attention and enjoyment, illustrating the deep connections between reading, learning, and emotional well-being.

A so-called "reading schedule" should allow room for adaptations based on your child's interests and moods. Too much structure can lead to resistance, leaving children feeling as if reading is a chore. Instead, a flexible approach can make reading an adventure, encouraging exploration and emotional growth in ways that rigid instruction can't achieve. After all, children need to perceive reading as a fun, fulfilling way to engage with the world. This sense of joy leads naturally to a thirst for knowledge.

It's vital to introduce a variety of reading materials that include fiction, nonfiction, poetry, and graphic novels, to name a few. This range serves to engage different aspects of cognitive and emotional processing in children. While fiction often strengthens empathy and ethics by involving children emotionally, non-fiction piques curiosity about the real world, sparking a hunger for knowledge. Both are integral to holistic cognitive development.

By achieving a balanced reading regimen, we can pave the way for children to develop robust cognitive capabilities and emotional intelligence. These children not only gain knowledge but also become adept at navigating the complexity of human emotions. They learn to appreciate different perspectives and horrors, to make informed decisions, and to connect meaningfully with others. The ultimate goal of harnessing reading as a tool for mental and emotional growth should be to develop well-rounded, emotionally intelligent individuals who cherish learning throughout their lives.

In conclusion, the delicate interplay between structure and free play in reading activities can have transformative effects on a child's cognitive and emotional development. We should strive to provide supportive environments that adapt to individual needs while encouraging both discipline and spontaneity in reading practices. Empowering children with such a balanced approach ensures not only adept readers but also resilient, empathetic, and critical thinkers.

Chapter 8: Managing Stress and Emotional Well-being

In today's fast-paced world, children and teens often encounter stressors that can impact their mental health and cognitive development. It's crucial to equip them with tools that build resilience and emotional well-being. Stress activates the brain's fight or flight response, which, if not managed, can interfere with their ability to learn and regulate emotions (Lupien et al., 2009). Encouraging healthy emotional regulation techniques, such as positive self-talk and structured problem-solving, can help children learn to navigate challenging emotions with more confidence (Gross, 2015). Additionally, fostering environments that emphasize positive social interactions and support networks plays a critical role in emotional development (Cacioppo et al., 2011). Mindfulness practices, including meditation and breathing exercises, have been shown to reduce stress levels and improve focus and emotional regulation. By integrating these practices into daily routines, caregivers can support children's emotional growth, helping them to face life's hurdles with a balanced mind and a resilient spirit.

The Brain's Response to Stress in Kids & Teens

Understanding how a child's brain responds to stress is crucial for anyone involved in their upbringing. Stress, unfortunately, is an inevitable part of life, but how it impacts children and teenagers is markedly different from adults. This difference stems largely from the fact that kids' brains are still developing, and crucial regions, including those involved in managing stress, emotions, and decision-making, are not yet fully matured.

When a child encounters stress, be it from school, social dynamics, or environmental pressures, the brain's immediate reaction involves the hypothalamic-pituitary-adrenal (HPA) axis. This system is responsible for producing cortisol, often termed the "stress hormone," and is crucial in managing our stress responses. In children, an elevated level of cortisol over prolonged periods can impair cognitive functions and emotional regulation (Gunnar & Quevedo, 2007). It's essential for caregivers to recognize this biological response to mitigate potential negative impacts.

The prefrontal cortex, pivotal for cognitive processes such as planning, attention, and emotion regulation, is among the last regions to fully develop in the brain. This delay in maturation is one reason why adolescents can struggle with managing stress and emotional upheaval effectively. It often results in heightened emotional responses and difficulties in concentration during stressful times (Casey et al., 2008). Supporting a child through these periods can involve strategies that ground them, offer reassurance, and allow space for emotional expression.

Repeated exposure to stress without adequate coping mechanisms can lead to long-term changes in the brain. Chronic stress can alter both the structure and function of brain areas related to decision-making and emotional regulation. For example, the amygdala, responsible for processing emotions like fear and pleasure, can become hyperactive, leading children to perceive threats more readily than calm situations (McEwen, 2007). This altered perception can be challenging for children but can be modulated with structured interventions.

One of the significant roles of parents, teachers, and caregivers is to provide a protective buffer against these stressors. Constructive intervention strategies could include fostering a supportive environment, promoting healthy relationships, and encouraging positive social interactions. Emotional validation, where a child's feelings are acknowledged and respected, provides a safe platform to explore those emotions without fear of reprimand or misunderstanding. This approach not only aids in stress management but also develops trust and empathy.

Moreover, mindfulness practices such as meditation and breathing exercises have been shown to significantly reduce stress and its psychological burden on the brain (Zenner et al., 2014). Introducing these techniques early helps children manage stress and equips them with lifelong skills for emotional regulation. Activities like yoga and tai chi might also offer dual benefits by promoting physical health alongside mental balance. Such practices are powerful tools to cultivate resilience.

Importantly, the context in which stress arises must be considered. Stress from household instability, for instance, might induce a stronger response compared to minor school challenges. Recognizing environmental stressors and addressing them, either by improving the home environment or school conditions, is key. Teachers and school administrators play a critical role here, as supportive educational environments contribute significantly to a child's ability to handle stress constructively.

In adolescence, peer relationships often become a significant source of both stress and support. Social connections can serve as a buffer against stress by providing emotional support and shared experiences. Programs that build social skills, such as group activities or team sports, not only improve peer interactions but also teach children the value of collaboration and shared goals. Positive social environments can mitigate the stress response by framing stress as a shared, not isolated, experience.

Let's not forget that diet and sleep play foundational roles in how stress affects the brain. Malnutrition or poor sleep can exacerbate stress and its effects on the brain, creating a vicious cycle that impairs learning and emotional stability. Establishing routines around nutrition and sleep can significantly reduce stress levels in children and teens. Ensuring a balanced diet rich in brain-boosting nutrients, adequate hydration, and a consistent sleep schedule creates an optimal environment for healthy brain development (Mindell & Owens, 2015).

In conclusion, recognizing and addressing stress in children and adolescents is not just about managing immediate symptoms but about fostering an environment that supports emotional and cognitive development. Tools and strategies such as mindfulness, emotional validation, nutritious diets, and supportive relationships are essential. By understanding the unique ways in which stress affects young brains, parents, teachers, and caregivers can better support their children, guiding them to build resilience and thrive in the face of life's inevitable challenges.

Emotional Regulation Techniques for Children

Understanding and managing emotions is crucial in children's development. It lays the foundation for healthy emotional well-being as they grow. While children naturally experience a range of emotions, it's the ability to regulate these emotions effectively that can alter their social interactions, academic performance, and general happiness. Implementing strategies for emotional regulation helps them develop resilience and adaptability, key life skills in our dynamic world.

At the heart of emotional regulation are self-awareness and understanding. When children begin to recognize and label their emotions, they can start understanding the causes and consequences. Educators and caregivers can facilitate this by helping children articulate emotions through language, using simple terms like "happy," "sad," or "angry" for younger kids, and introducing more nuanced emotions like "frustrated" or "disappointed" as they age. This builds an emotional vocabulary, which is vital for effective communication and emotional processing (Gottman et al., 1996).

One of the simplest yet most effective emotional regulation techniques is deep breathing. This method helps children to pause, take control, and calm their physiological responses to stressors. Encouraging children to take deep, slow breaths when they feel upset can significantly reduce the intensity of their emotions. Breathing exercises can easily be transformed into fun activities or games, where children blow bubbles or pretend they're balloons, allowing them to engage with the practice in a playful manner.

Another essential aspect is the role of physical activity in managing emotions. Regular physical activity not only contributes to physical health but also to mental well-being. Movement can release endorphins, which are natural mood lifters, and reduce cortisol levels, the hormone associated with stress. For children, activities like dancing, playing tag, or practicing yoga can be particularly effective. Yoga, in particular, has been shown to improve self-regulation, mood, and even cognitive performance in children (Stueck & Gloeckner, 2005).

Teaching problem-solving skills is another crucial component in emotional regulation. Often, emotional dysregulation in children can stem from feelings of helplessness or confusion in particular situations. By equipping children with problem-solving skills, caregivers and teachers can enhance their ability to navigate challenges, reduce stress, and foster a sense of autonomy. This involves guiding children through a process of identifying the problem, brainstorming possible solutions, evaluating the options, and then trying out the selected solution. Over time, this process strengthens their confidence and resilience.

Additionally, modeling emotional regulation is indispensable. Children learn a great deal by observing the adults around them. When adults demonstrate healthy ways of managing emotions—like remaining calm during stressful situations or verbally processing their emotions—children are more likely to mimic these behaviors. Encouraging open discussions about feelings within the family or classroom setting can also normalize emotional expression and equip children with strategies to manage their emotions effectively (Bandura, 1986).

Some children may benefit particularly from mindfulness and meditation practices. These techniques encourage present-moment awareness and foster emotional regulation by helping children observe their thoughts and feelings without immediate reaction. Mindfulness exercises can be simple and brief, such as focusing on the sensation of their breath or listening intently to the sounds in the room. Consistent practice of mindfulness has been associated with improved emotional regulation, attention, and social skills (Semple et al., 2010).

A nurturing environment that emphasizes security and acceptance is pivotal for effective emotional regulation. Children who feel safe are more willing to communicate their emotions and experiment with different regulation techniques. Creating an atmosphere where emotions are not judged but understood is essential. This includes providing children with the assurance that it's okay to make mistakes and feel different things at different times.

Reward systems can be strategically used to encourage emotional regulation efforts in children. Positive reinforcement, such as praise or reward for using a regulation strategy effectively, can motivate children to keep using these techniques. It's important, however, to focus not just on the outcome but the process, valuing their effort in attempting to manage their emotions.

Technology can also be leveraged to support emotional regulation in children. Various apps and digital tools are available to help guide children through breathing exercises, meditations, or identify emotions.

These tools often present strategies in engaging formats—stories, games, or animated sequences—that resonate with children and maintain their interest.

In summary, fostering emotional regulation in children involves a multi-faceted approach that blends understanding, practice, modeling, and technology. While it's natural for children to struggle with emotions at times, these strategies provide the tools they need to navigate their feelings healthily and effectively. By equipping them with these skills early on, we empower them to handle life's challenges with confidence and resilience, paving the way for a well-rounded, emotionally balanced adulthood.

The Importance of Positive Social Interactions & Support

To truly manage stress and bolster emotional well-being in children, the role of positive social interactions and support networks can't be overstated. At its core, human development is defined by relationships—be it with family, friends, teachers, or peers. These interactions shape how young minds perceive and engage with the world, setting the foundation for their future cognitive and emotional landscapes. The science behind it is substantial: positive social interactions can trigger the release of oxytocin, often dubbed the "feel-good" hormone, which helps buffer stress and enhance mood (Cacioppo et al., 2014).

Consider the transformative power of a warm greeting or a genuine smile. These seemingly simple gestures foster feelings of safety and acceptance, establishing a nurturing environment where children can thrive. Such interactions can improve a child's self-esteem, encourage resilience, and buffer against the adverse effects of stress. In educational settings, students who perceive strong support from teachers are more motivated and engaged, which in turn enhances their academic performance and overall well-being (Wentzel, 2012).

But what is it about these social interactions that make them so pivotal in supporting emotional well-being? It's the sense of belonging and acceptance they foster. When a child feels valued within a group, whether in a classroom, family, or peer setting, their emotional resilience naturally strengthens. This indicates not only how much children learn from the content of interactions but also from the emotional context in which they occur.

Building these connections requires intentional effort from adults. Parents, teachers, and caregivers play crucial roles in modeling positive interactions. They must create environments where children feel comfortable expressing themselves without fear of judgment. Notably, the practice of active listening can't be ignored. When a child knows they're truly heard, it validates their feelings and experiences, helping them develop self-worth and emotional intelligence.

The impact of peer relationships on stress management is particularly significant during adolescence. Adolescents often turn to peers for support more than any other age group. These peer ties offer unique opportunities for social learning, where mutual support can lead to stronger coping mechanisms and improved stress management strategies (Prinstein & Giletta, 2016). However, it's crucial to guide children in nurturing healthy peer interactions and recognizing the signs of toxic relationships, which could harm their emotional development.

Furthermore, fostering positive social interactions requires a balance between structured activities and free play. While structured activities can facilitate teamwork and cooperation, unstructured play allows children to develop social skills organically. This blend can teach children not only how to initiate interactions but also how to navigate complex social dynamics, such as conflict resolution and empathy.

Community support can enhance the resilience of both children and adults. Teachers and parents working together, for instance, can create a supportive network that amplifies their efforts. Community programs focusing on group activities, such as team sports or art workshops, provide a platform for children to build their social skills in diverse environments. Such programs highlight the community's role in providing additional layers of support and engagement vital for children's growth.

Moreover, the emphasis on positive reinforcement rather than punitive measures can lead to more sustainable outcomes in emotional health. Encouraging positive behaviors through praise and rewards helps cultivate a supportive atmosphere. Even in disciplinary situations, constructive feedback should be aimed at understanding and growth rather than punishment (Dweck, 2007). This not only reduces stress but also aligns children's behavior with desirable social norms.

Despite the clear benefits, there are challenges, too. The digital age presents unique tests, where online interactions can sometimes replace face-to-face communication. While technology offers vast avenues for connection, it is crucial for caregivers to ensure that these connections are genuinely supportive and do not isolate children further. Encouraging balanced screen use with mindful interaction can help preserve the quality of social support offered by digital means.

Finally, encouraging positive social interactions involves celebrating diversity and teaching acceptance. Exposure to diverse groups enhances children's social competence and cultural understanding, allowing them to function well in an increasingly interconnected world. This involves educating children about compassion, empathy, and the acceptance of differences, which equips them to build varied yet positive social relationships.

Ultimately, the presence of supportive social networks is not just beneficial but foundational to managing stress and fostering emotional well-being in children. These networks offer a buffer against life's stressors and serve as a springboard for emotional and cognitive growth. As adults committed to nurturing the next generation, it is our role to facilitate these connections, ensuring that every child has the support they need to flourish.

The Impact of Mindfulness, Meditation, and Breathing Exercises

In the ever-evolving journey of childhood and adolescence, stress can often appear as an uninvited guest. While some stress can act as a motivator, chronic stress is another story altogether. Prolonged stress affects not only a child's emotional well-being but also their cognitive function. It's here that mindfulness, meditation, and breathing exercises come into play, offering a buffer that aids in managing this stress effectively. These practices are more than just trends; they are rooted in scientific principles with tangible benefits for the developing brain (Tang et al., 2015).

Mindfulness, at its core, is about being present in the moment without judgment. When children engage in mindfulness practices, they learn to ground themselves and move away from automatic reactions to stress. This simple act of paying attention can foster deeper awareness and a more profound connection with their thoughts and emotions. A study by Schonert-Reichl et al. (2015) highlighted how students who participated in mindfulness training showed improvements in empathy, perspective-taking, and emotional resilience. These emotional skills are foundational to well-rounded cognitive development and significant in navigating social dynamics.

Meditation, in conjunction with mindfulness, provides a powerful duo in combating stress. Meditation exercises for children aren't about achieving a zen-like state but rather about cultivating a state of calm focus and relaxation. Regular practice helps quiet mental chatter and activate the brain areas responsible for emotional regulation and attention (Luders et al., 2009). Through meditation, children can enhance their attention span, gain emotional clarity, and develop a stronger sense of self-awareness. Encouraging children to engage in brief periods of meditation can substantially enhance their emotional health, a critical component of holistic brain development.

Breathing exercises complement mindfulness and meditation by offering quick and effective stress-relief solutions. Simple techniques, such as slow, deep breathing, can lower heart rate and reduce anxiety by signaling the brain to shift from a stress response to a relaxation response. When children practice these techniques, they not only calm themselves but also increase their capacity to cope with future stressors. These exercises act as grounding tools, especially useful in high-stress situations such as exams or conflict resolutions. By teaching children how to control their breath, we empower them with a tool that's always available, much like a mental first-aid kit.

The integration of these practices in a young person's life can lead to a more focused and balanced individual. It doesn't require a significant time commitment. Even a few minutes of daily practice can lead to notable changes. Schools and caregivers can foster environments where these exercises become routine, possibly incorporating them into daily schedules or classroom activities. As children become more adept at these practices, they develop a toolbox of skills for managing stress throughout their lives.

However, it's essential to introduce these practices in a way that's engaging and age-appropriate. Younger children might enjoy guided meditations with imaginative storytelling elements, while teenagers might appreciate more straightforward techniques that they can practice independently. The key is to make mindfulness, meditation, and breathing exercises an enjoyable and integral part of their daily routine rather than a chore. By doing so, we not only support their emotional and cognitive development but also lay a foundation for a lifelong habit of self-care.

In conclusion, the introduction of mindfulness, meditation, and breathing exercises into the lives of children and adolescents has profound implications for their stress management and emotional well-being. By equipping them with these practices, we offer more than just a tool for today; we gift them a habit of a lifetime that supports a balanced mind and a resilient spirit. It's a small investment with a potentially enormous return in forming emotionally intelligent, self-aware, and cognitively adept future adults.

Chapter 9: Screen Time – Finding the Right Balance

Navigating the digital age as a caregiver involves more than just setting time limits on devices; it requires a nuanced understanding of how screens impact young minds. Striking the right balance in screen time is pivotal not merely for protecting children from overstimulation but also for leveraging technology to enhance cognitive and emotional growth. Too much screen exposure, especially before bedtime, can disrupt sleep patterns and hinder emotional regulation (Cain & Gradisar, 2010). On the flip side, curated educational apps and programs can foster learning and critical thinking if used appropriately (Hirsh-Pasek et al., 2015). Setting age-appropriate boundaries is crucial—this means understanding that a preschooler's needs and screen consumption will differ significantly from that of a teenager. Encouraging breaks, incorporating physical activities, and opting for interactive over passive content are key strategies in cultivating a healthy media environment (Straker et al., 2017). The goal isn't to demonize screens but rather to integrate them mindfully into daily routines, creating a space where they contribute positively to a child's developmental journey.

The Pros and Cons of Digital Devices for Cognitive Development

In today's digital age, children are constantly surrounded by various forms of technology. From smartphones to tablets and computers, digital devices are now integral to their daily lives. As parents, teachers, and caregivers, it's crucial to understand how these devices influence cognitive development. There are both advantages and challenges associated with digital device use, and striking the right balance is essential.

On the positive side, digital devices can provide significant educational benefits. With a multitude of educational apps and online resources, they offer opportunities for learning that were not available in the past. These tools can cater to different learning styles, providing interactive and engaging content that can enhance cognitive skills such as problem-solving, critical thinking, and creativity. For instance, apps designed for learning new languages or improving math skills can be both effective and enjoyable, motivating children to engage in educational activities outside of school hours (Hirsh-Pasek et al., 2015).

Moreover, digital devices can enhance cognitive flexibility by providing dynamic environments where children must adapt to new rules or challenges. Video games, for example, often require players to think quickly, strategize, and make decisions under pressure, all of which can contribute to cognitive development. Such games can improve hand-eye coordination, spatial awareness, and reaction times, which play a role in brain development as well (Granic et al., 2014).

Despite these benefits, there are also several concerns regarding the overuse of digital devices. One of the most significant issues is the potential impact on attention spans. The fast-paced and highly stimulating nature of many digital applications can condition children to expect constant sensory input, which might hinder their ability to focus on less stimulating tasks such as reading or homework. Some studies suggest that excessive screen time can lead to attention disorders, although more research is needed to establish a direct causal link (Christakis, 2009).

Digital device use may also affect memory and learning processes. In many cases, the use of technology can become a replacement for critical thinking and memory retention. With access to information at the touch of a button, children might rely too heavily on devices for answers, which can limit their ability to store and recall information independently. This reliance may impact their long-term cognitive development, as the act of memorizing and retrieving information is crucial in building strong neural connections.

Another important aspect to consider is the effect of digital devices on emotional regulation. Exposure to online content that is not age-appropriate can foster anxiety, stress, and other emotional challenges. Moreover, the pressure of maintaining a certain image on social media platforms can contribute to low self-esteem and issues related to peer comparison. Such emotional stressors can interfere with cognitive functions and impede a child's ability to learn effectively.

Given these pros and cons, how should parents and educators approach digital device usage in a way that supports cognitive development while minimizing potential harm? One strategy is to foster an environment where digital device use is balanced with other activities. Encouraging activities such as outdoor play, reading physical books, and engaging in creative projects can provide counterbalance to screen time. This holistic approach ensures that children develop a wide range of skills that are not solely dependent on digital technology.

Setting clear and consistent boundaries around screen time is also crucial. Limiting the use of digital devices to certain hours of the day, especially avoiding screen use before bedtime, can help mitigate negative effects. This limitation can prevent disruptions in sleep patterns, which are vital for cognitive and emotional recovery and growth. Collaboratively creating a family media plan that defines acceptable uses for digital devices can promote healthy habits and self-regulation, aiding in the development of executive functions in children.

Additionally, adults can guide children in selecting high-quality educational content and cultivating critical media literacy. Teaching children to question the information they encounter and understand the difference between educational content and passive entertainment can enhance their analytical skills. By actively engaging with children during their digital interactions, parents and educators can provide context and encourage discussion about the content being consumed.

In summary, digital devices present both opportunities and challenges for cognitive development in children. By wisely integrating technology into children's lives and maintaining a balanced approach, we can leverage the benefits while minimizing potential downsides. As always, the role of caring adults is pivotal in guiding children through their interactions with technology, ensuring they develop into well-rounded individuals.

How Screens Impact Attention, Memory, and Emotional Regulation

In this digital age, screens are ubiquitous in children's lives, posing unique challenges to their attention, memory, and emotional regulation. The rapid pace at which technology has integrated into daily routines, from educational resources to leisure activities, necessitates a thoughtful examination of its impact on young minds. While digital devices offer several educational benefits, their influence on cognitive and emotional development requires careful navigation to ensure healthy usage patterns.

Attention, a crucial cognitive function, is often the first to show signs of strain in a screen-dense environment. The constant shifts in stimuli, from flashing lights to rapid changes in imagery, can lead to shortened attention spans. Research indicates that frequent exposure to digital media may condition children to expect high levels of stimulation, making it difficult for them to focus on tasks that demand sustained mental effort (Christakis, 2019). This phenomenon is known as "attentional fatigue," which reduces the capacity to concentrate over extended periods, a skill essential for academic success and daily life (Hale et al., 2018).

Memory, another vital component of cognitive development, also faces challenges in a world filled with screens. The oversaturation of information can overwhelm working memory, the system responsible for holding and processing short-term data. Children might struggle to transfer knowledge from working memory to long-term memory, essential for learning and retention (Temple et al., 2019). Furthermore, the reliance on digital devices for information retrieval may discourage the development of internal memory systems, as children may opt to "Google" answers rather than recall from memory. This dependency can hinder the ability to engage in critical thinking and problem-solving, skills crucial in both educational settings and real-world scenarios.

Emotional regulation is no less affected by screen exposure. Emotional skills develop through real-world interactions, where facial expressions, tone, and body language play vital roles. However, excessive screen time can limit these face-to-face interactions, leaving children less equipped to recognize and manage emotions effectively. Social media, in particular, introduces complexities such as cyberbullying and the pressure of idealized portrayals, which can distort self-image and mental health (Anderson & Jiang, 2018). Studies suggest that higher levels of screen time correlate with increased rates of anxiety and depression in children and adolescents, highlighting the urgent need for monitoring and moderating digital consumption (Twenge & Campbell, 2018).

Nonetheless, not all screen interactions are detrimental; their impact largely depends on the nature of the content and the context of usage. Educational content, when interactive and age-appropriate, can enhance learning and engagement. Programs designed to build language skills or encourage critical thinking offer potential benefits, especially when combined with parental involvement. It's the difference between passive consumption and active engagement that often determines the outcome. Active engagement with educational material can stimulate cognitive processes, reinforcing skills learned in traditional environments (Wartella et al., 2016).

Addressing the effects of screens on children involves striking a delicate balance. Establishing guidelines that prioritize high-quality content and set healthy boundaries around usage can mediate negative influences. Integrating screen-free periods in daily routines encourages alternative activities, such as outdoor play and reading, which are essential for holistic development. Encouraging children to participate in games and activities that require critical thinking, collaboration, and creativity helps foster skills that screens alone cannot enhance.

Moreover, role-modeling healthy screen habits is crucial. Children often mimic adult behaviors, so cultivating family norms around device use can positively influence their habits. Creating tech-free zones or times, such as during meals or before bedtime, can promote more meaningful engagement with surroundings and facilitate better sleep hygiene, further supporting overall cognitive and emotional health.

Another vital strategy is teaching digital literacy. Educating children about the purpose and consequences of their digital interactions empowers them to make informed choices. Open communication about the content they encounter online and its potential impacts can demystify digital experiences, reducing anxiety and enhancing resilience.

Likewise, interdisciplinary approaches involving educators, healthcare practitioners, and parents can provide comprehensive strategies to manage screen time effectively. Incorporating technology into structured educational environments with set objectives and outcomes ensures that screens serve as tools for enhancement rather than distraction. Collaborative efforts can help devise adaptable frameworks that evolve with technological advancements and changing societal norms.

Technology isn't inherently harmful. When used mindfully, it can be a powerful tool for learning and connection. The challenge lies in crafting environments that allow children to experience the world both through and beyond screens. With intentionality and awareness, screens can coexist with traditional methods of learning and interaction, enriching rather than hindering cognitive and emotional development.

In conclusion, as the role of screens in children's lives continues to expand, understanding their impacts on attention, memory, and emotional regulation becomes increasingly essential. Empowering children to navigate their digital worlds thoughtfully can safeguard their cognitive and emotional well-being while preparing them for future challenges and opportunities in an ever-evolving landscape.

Educational vs. Passive Entertainment Content

As parents, teachers, or caregivers, one of the most significant decisions we face is how to manage children's screen time effectively. In today's digital landscape, not all content is created equal, and differentiating between educational and passive entertainment is critical to supporting cognitive and emotional development. While screen time often gets a bad rap, it's essential to acknowledge that when used wisely, digital content can offer substantial educational benefits (Domine, 2022).

Educational content is designed to engage children actively and requires their involvement in learning processes. Think of interactive apps that teach math or science concepts, digital storybooks encouraging reading, or language-learning programs. These types of content can enhance problem-solving skills, improve cognitive functions, and promote creativity (Hirsh-Pasek et al., 2015). Moreover, they often incorporate elements that require active participation, such as solving puzzles or making decisions, which can translate to improved executive functions such as working memory and cognitive flexibility.

On the flip side, passive entertainment, though not devoid of value entirely, often involves content like non-interactive TV shows or videos that do not demand mental engagement from viewers. While these can serve as a form of relaxation or provide a sense of downtime, excessive exposure might contribute to increased sedentary behavior and reduced time for more physically active pursuits (Pagani et al., 2019). In a balanced screen-time regimen, entertainment has its place but should be moderated to ensure it doesn't overshadow educational opportunities and physical activities.

Striking the right balance between educational content and passive entertainment requires a keen understanding of your child's unique needs and interests. Consider their age and developmental stage; younger children may find more value in simple interactive games or story apps, while older kids might benefit from content that challenges their analytical thinking and problem-solving abilities. Integrative content that combines entertainment with educational elements — edutainment — can also be a valuable tool.

Setting guidelines is beneficial. Encourage children to participate in choosing educational programs and games, fostering a collaborative approach that builds autonomy over their media choices. It's essential, however, to maintain awareness without crossing into micromanagement. Trust in the process that promotes self-regulation can empower kids to select content serving their developmental goals (Roseberry et al., 2014).

As technology evolves, so do opportunities for learning. Virtual reality, for instance, offers multisensory experiences that can make complex subjects like science and history more tangible and immersive. These innovations enable children to visualize and interact with information in ways that textbooks and traditional learning environments might not (Dede, 2009). Such experiences underscore the importance of leveraging technology to unlock new learning dimensions.

The content should not threaten the balance of family and social life. Research indicates that excessive screen time, particularly passive consumption, can negatively impact children's social skills and emotional intelligence. Face-to-face interactions are irreplaceable for developing empathy, communication skills, and emotional awareness (Uhls, 2014). As a result, creating media-rich environments that don't overshadow valuable real-world interactions is crucial.

Furthermore, understanding the impact of excessive passive screen time on mental health is vital. A growing body of evidence points towards potential risks for anxiety and depression, primarily owing to its association with sedentary behavior and reduced physical activity (Twenge & Campbell, 2018). Balancing educational digital content with active play and ensuring regular physical activity can mitigate these risks and contribute positively to overall well-being.

Recognizing the individual differences among children is also crucial. Some might thrive with more digital content, whereas others benefit from minimal exposure. Engaging in open conversations with children about their media consumption preferences and behaviors is instrumental in tailoring an approach that aligns with their interests and developmental needs (Radesky & Christakis, 2016).

Educational content extends beyond academic purposes; it can foster emotional intelligence and resilience. Digital stories and games portraying moral dilemmas or emotional challenges can provide safe spaces for children to explore their feelings, learn coping strategies, and develop empathy (Greenberg & Reiner, 2016). Introducing such content thoughtfully can nurture emotional growth alongside cognitive development.

Lastly, setting an example through mindful screen use is paramount. Parents and caregivers serve as role models; children learn by observing adult behaviors. Demonstrating a balanced approach to media consumption — prioritizing quality content and integrating screen-free periods — reinforces the intended message and encourages children to adopt healthy media habits.

Balancing educational and passive entertainment content is an ongoing process. By engaging in continual dialogue, setting clear expectations, and remaining vigilant about content quality, we can ensure that children's screen time supports their cognitive and emotional growth. The ultimate aim is not just to limit screen time but to enrich it, transforming digital interactions into powerful educational experiences that prepare children for the complexities of the world.

How Much is Too Much? Setting Age-Appropriate Limits

Finding the right balance with screen time can be a challenging endeavor for parents, teachers, and caregivers who aim to nurture children's cognitive and emotional development. With technology becoming an integrated part of everyday life, it's crucial to understand how much screen time is too much and how to set age-appropriate limits. In the era of digital advancements, children are more exposed to screens than ever before, affecting their attention, memory, and overall well-being. Establishing these limits isn't just about control; it's about empowering children to maximize their development in a digital world while safeguarding their mental and physical health.

Children's brains develop rapidly, particularly within the first few years of life, and this is a time when they are particularly susceptible to environmental influences, including screen exposure. According to the American Academy of Pediatrics, children younger than 18 months should discourage any screen usage, except for video chatting (AAP, 2016). From 18 to 24 months, if you choose to introduce digital media, it should be high-quality programming that you and your children can view together. It's not only about the content but also about engaging in the experience with them.

For children aged two to five, screen time should be limited to one hour per day of high-quality programming (AAP, 2016). This limit ensures that screens aren't taking the place of critical developmental activities like active play and interaction with caregivers. During these formative years, children learn best through unstructured play, hands-on experiences, and social interactions. These activities are vital for language development, problem-solving skills, and emotional regulation, which can all be hindered by excessive screen time.

As children grow into school-aged kids, screen habits become more challenging to manage due to educational demands and social influences. It's essential to maintain a balance that allows children to benefit from technology while not succumbing to its pitfalls. For ages six and older, parents are advised to place consistent limits on screen time, ensuring it does not interfere with sleep, physical activity, and other essential health behaviors ("Children and Media Tips from the American Academy of Pediatrics," 2016). Co-viewing, co-playing, and discussing the content can enhance understanding and improve communication, making screen time more beneficial.

The discussion around screen time also needs to change as children advance into their teenage years. During adolescence, there's a growing need for autonomy, but also an increasing risk of screen misuse related to social media and gaming. The focus should shift towards helping teenagers self-regulate their screen time, emphasizing the importance of personal responsibility and critical thinking about the media they consume. Engaging teens in creating a "family technology plan" that includes no screens during meals or before bed can be an effective strategy for fostering a healthy relationship with technology (AAP, 2016).

While evaluating screen time, it's important to consider not just the quantity but also the quality of the content consumed. Educational and interactive media can be considerably more enriching than passive screen consumption. Shows and games that promote active engagement, problem-solving, or creativity can be valuable tools that complement learning and development, rather than detracting from it. It's essential for caregivers to vet content thoroughly and steer children toward media that aligns with developmental goals and values.

Moreover, screen time should not act as a substitute for essential life experiences. Regular breaks from screens encourage children to engage with their environment, fostering creativity and imagination through traditional play. Interactions with family, friends, and peers provide opportunities for developing social skills and emotional intelligence—skills that are indispensable in navigating the challenges of the modern world.

Adults must also model healthy screen habits, as children often emulate the behaviors they observe. By setting personal limits and demonstrating balanced media use, caregivers can reinforce the importance of moderation and encourage healthier patterns. Technology should serve as a bridge to achieving development goals, not a barrier.

It's also relevant to address the potential risks associated with excessive screen use, such as sleep disturbances. Screen exposure, particularly before bedtime, can interfere with sleep quality by suppressing melatonin, a hormone crucial for sleep regulation (Hale & Guan, 2015). To mitigate such effects, establish a screen-free period at least an hour before bedtime. This simple adjustment can significantly enhance a child's sleep quality and overall health.

Lastly, collaboration between parents, educators, and health professionals may be needed to ensure that screen time recommendations are feasible and context-appropriate. Each child's environmental context and individual needs vary; thus, a flexible approach in determining screen time limits can be beneficial.

The key lies in staying informed, understanding the intricacies of screen time impacts, and setting boundaries that respect children's needs to explore and learn in a digital world while ensuring they don't miss out on the hands-on experiences essential for their growth. Balance is imperative to fostering an environment where children can thrive both online and offline, laying the groundwork for a healthier and well-rounded future.

Nighttime Screen Use & Its Effects on Sleep & Focus

In today's digital age, it's become commonplace for screens to populate every corner of our lives, from smartphones to tablets and laptops. For children and adolescents, this often translates to extensive screen exposure, particularly in the evening hours, which can significantly disrupt sleep patterns and focus. Understanding the subtle and not-so-subtle ways in which nighttime screen use affects young minds is vital for parents, teachers, and caregivers aiming to promote optimal cognitive and emotional development.

One of the most well-documented effects of evening screen exposure is its impact on sleep. The blue light emitted by most screens suppresses the secretion of melatonin, the hormone responsible for regulating sleep-wake cycles (Cain & Gradisar, 2010). This suppression can lead to difficulties in falling asleep, reduced sleep duration, and altered sleep quality. Youngsters who use screens just before bed may find themselves tossing and turning, which in turn affects their daytime alertness and ability to concentrate.

Sleep deprivation in children isn't a minor inconvenience. It's a critical issue, as insufficient sleep can impair attention, working memory, and even decision-making skills. Moreover, chronic sleep loss has been linked to a host of negative outcomes, including mood swings, increased stress levels, and a decrease in academic performance (Owens et al., 2016). For children, the time spent on a screen late at night doesn't just replace sleep; it compromises the entire following day's activities due to reduced cognitive and emotional functioning.

It's not just the blue light that's detrimental; the content on these screens often plays a role too. Engaging in stimulating or emotionally charged activities, like playing a video game or watching an exciting show, can elevate adrenaline levels and keep the mind active when it should be winding down. The pre-bedtime period should ideally be one of relaxation—a time to transition from the day's hustle and bustle into a restful night (Hale & Guan, 2015).

In an age of digital convenience, setting clear boundaries around screen use isn't just beneficial—it's necessary. Establishing media curfews, which involve powering down all electronic devices at least an hour before bedtime, can help facilitate better sleep hygiene. Instead of screen time, families might consider engaging in calming activities such as reading a book or listening to soothing music. These practices not only pave the way for improved sleep quality but also allow children to wind down effectively.

Moreover, it's essential to foster environments that encourage healthier media consumption habits. This could involve integrating educational tools that teach children about the effects of screen use on sleep and focus. Schools and communities can play a pivotal role by promoting awareness and providing resources that help children and parents understand the direct correlation between screen exposure and its effects on sleep and concentration.

The ongoing development of children's brains makes them particularly vulnerable to the ramifications of poor screen habits. Thus, supporting healthy screen time management is akin to investing in their future cognitive and emotional resilience. By ensuring a balance between technology use and necessary rest, caregivers can significantly enhance children's overall brain health and emotional well-being.

Lastly, it's crucial to remember that these guidelines aren't about demonizing technology. Instead, they're about cultivating an environment where technology is used responsibly and thoughtfully. This can empower children to develop healthy digital habits that will benefit them throughout their lives, providing a strong foundation for academic success and socio-emotional health.

Encouraging Healthy Media Consumption Habits

In today's digital age, screens are ubiquitous, and media consumption has woven itself into the very fabric of daily life. As such, finding a healthy balance in media consumption, especially for children, is more critical than ever. The objective is not to vilify digital tools but to create an environment where technology serves as a beneficial component of a child's development rather than a detriment. Understanding the impact of media requires an approach that integrates empathy and science while offering actionable strategies for parents, teachers, and caregivers.

Parents might feel overwhelmed by the vast array of media options available. It's important to first establish guidelines that align with your family's values. Begin by creating a media plan that balances screen time with other essential activities like physical play, reading, and face-to-face interactions. According to the American Academy of Pediatrics, setting consistent limits on media use is crucial for children's wellness ("AAP," 2016). These limits should vary according to the child's age and developmental needs, emphasizing how quality content can promote learning and creativity while avoiding passive consumption.

When it comes to selecting appropriate content, parents should consider the pedagogical value of media. Media that fosters critical thinking and problem-solving offers more developmental benefits than passive entertainment. Educational programs, interactive applications, and documentaries can be harnessed to stimulate curiosity and intellectual growth. However, the engagement should be monitored to ensure children are critically interacting with content rather than passively absorbing it.

Encouraging active participation from the child is vital. Use media as a springboard for conversation. For example, after viewing a documentary or playing an educational game together, discuss what was learned and explore deeper insights. This not only enhances cognitive development but strengthens emotional connections. Sharing media experiences as a family can turn screen time from an isolating activity into an inclusive, enriching one.

The pervasive nature of screens has also necessitated discussions about attention management and self-regulation. Excessive media consumption can fracture attention spans and is often associated with increased distractibility in children. The design of many digital platforms inherently promotes constant stimulation, making it essential to implement mindful viewing practices. Mindfulness, when integrated with screen use, encourages children to be aware of their engagement intentions, fostering more mindful, deliberate consumption.

Caregivers can model and teach emotional self-regulation strategies to counterbalance potential adverse effects of media exposure. Encouraging children to express and articulate their feelings about certain content can fortify emotional literacy. This literacy extends beyond the media and aids in managing daily emotional highs and lows—practicing self-regulation builds resilience and adaptability in various situations (Siegel, 2012).

In this era of potential overexposure to digital devices, reinforcing the joys of offline activities is equally crucial. Active breaks during media use can reduce screen fatigue and replenish cognitive resources. Suggest activities that require physical movement or creative output, such as drawing or playing an instrument. These activities are known to enhance neural integration, boosting both cognitive abilities and emotional health (Ratey & Hagerman, 2008).

Furthermore, the media's influence on social behavior cannot be overstated. Social skills develop when children engage in play and real-life interactions. Programs should not act as a surrogate for human contact. Encourage dialogues and social play to facilitate these important social learning experiences. It involves not just time management but intentional curation of experiences that balance digital interactions with physical world engagements.

Ultimately, creating healthy media consumption habits involves ongoing adaptation and communication. Stay informed about new platforms and their effects on developing brains, supported by scientific studies and expert advice. Regularly review and adjust media plans to reflect the child's evolving needs and any new insights emerging from research in developmental psychology ("AAP," 2016; Gentile et al., 2017).

For caregivers, partnering with children in their media consumption journey enables both autonomy and mindfulness in choices. Such collaboration encourages children to become discerning consumers of media, capable of distinguishing beneficial content from detrimental. The goal is not only to instill discipline but to empower children with the skills needed to navigate the digital world responsibly and effectively.

Chapter 10: Video Games & Digital Play – Boosting or Harming Brain Development?

Exploring the role of video games and digital play in children's lives is a complex yet essential aspect of modern parenting and education. On one hand, interactive games have shown potential in enhancing cognitive abilities such as decision-making, processing speed, and adaptability, which can significantly support brain development (Granic et al., 2014). Strategy-based and problem-solving games can serve as powerful tools for developing executive function and cognitive flexibility. However, there's a flip side to this digital engagement. Excessive gaming may lead to issues like dopamine overload, impacting focus and motivation adversely (Pontes & Griffiths, 2015). Additionally, prolonged gaming sessions can contribute to sleep disruptions, which are crucial for the brain's recovery cycle, potentially hindering emotional and cognitive health (Cain & Gradisar, 2010). Thus, it becomes imperative for caregivers to find a balanced approach. Encouraging a mix of digital play with outdoor physical activity, enforcing healthy gaming habits, and selecting games that bolster learning and emotional resilience can transform video gaming into a supportive element of one's developmental toolkit. By establishing boundaries and promoting diverse activities, adults can help leverage the positive aspects of video games while mitigating potential risks.

The Cognitive Benefits of Video Games & Interactive Digital Play

In recent years, there's been an ongoing debate amongst parents, educators, and researchers regarding the impact of video games and interactive digital play on children's cognitive development. While concerns about potential negative effects exist, numerous studies suggest that video games, when chosen and used appropriately, offer a variety of cognitive benefits that can significantly enhance brain development. Understanding these benefits allows us to make informed decisions that support children's cognitive and emotional growth.

One of the primary cognitive benefits of video games is their ability to enhance executive function, which includes skills like decision-making, processing speed, and adaptability. Fast-paced games, in particular, require players to swiftly analyze situations and respond to changing scenarios, thereby honing their ability to make quick decisions and think on their feet. This type of engagement fosters better problem-solving skills, as players must continually process information to achieve specific goals (Bavelier et al., 2012).

Strategy games offer additional cognitive benefits by compelling players to plan, strategize, and execute long-term goals. This genre of games promotes critical thinking and often mirrors real-world problem-solving processes. Players practice patience and foresight as they must predict opponents' moves and strategize accordingly—skills that are transferable to classroom settings and other real-life situations (Green & Bavelier, 2003).

Memory enhancement is another important cognitive benefit of digital play. Many video games require players to remember complex instructions, track characters' arcs, and recall past actions to progress. Such games, particularly role-playing games (RPGs), help sharpen working memory as players juggle multiple pieces of information to achieve objectives. These activities can enhance cognitive flexibility, which is crucial for learning multiple subjects and handling varying tasks effectively (Basak et al., 2008).

Beyond the cognitive skills enhancing mental processing, digital play can also support emotional resilience and stress relief. Engaging with games that offer a sense of achievement or provide immersive storytelling can help children develop persistence and emotional coping strategies. For instance, overcoming challenges in games can boost self-esteem and provide a safe space for managing frustration, mirroring life's hurdles in a controlled environment.

Despite these potential benefits, it remains crucial to approach video games with a balanced perspective. Not all video games are created equal, and excessive gaming can lead to detrimental outcomes, such as sleep disruption and decreased physical activity. Hence, identifying games that are educational or require cognitive engagement is important for maximizing the benefits while avoiding adverse effects (Gentile et al., 2009).

Educational and brain-training games have been specifically designed to enhance cognitive abilities like memory, attention, and processing speed. These types of digital play can supplement traditional learning and provide engaging ways for children to practice skills outside a classroom environment. However, it is essential to evaluate the effectiveness and scientific backing of these games, as not all are created with the same educational value (Oei & Patterson, 2013).

As with any tool, the key lies in moderation and informed selection. By choosing games that challenge the brain without overstimulating it, we can harness the cognitive benefits of digital play. Setting appropriate limits on gaming time ensures gaming remains a constructive part of a child's routine, rather than a dominant one. This balanced approach complements other brain-boosting activities, such as physical play and reading, providing a well-rounded environment for developing minds.

Ultimately, the cognitive benefits of video games and interactive digital play should be viewed holistically, balancing them with other critical elements of cognitive development, such as nutrition, sleep, and social interaction. By acknowledging and leveraging the positive aspects of digital play, caregivers can cultivate an environment that encourages cognitive growth and emotional well-being in children.

How Certain Games Improve Executive Function (Decision-Making, Processing Speed, Adaptability)

In recent years, video games have garnered attention for their potential to impact cognitive functions, challenging conventional views that gaming is merely a passive or even detrimental activity. Growing evidence suggests that specific types of video games can significantly enhance executive functions, particularly in the realms of decision-making, processing speed, and adaptability (Bediou et al., 2018). For many parents, teachers, and caregivers, understanding these potential benefits opens up new avenues for supporting children's cognitive and emotional development while harnessing the power of digital play.

Executive functions are the set of cognitive processes that enable goal-oriented behavior. These include the ability to process information quickly, adapt to new situations, and make informed decisions under conditions of uncertainty. Video games, particularly action games, have been found to enhance these capabilities by requiring players to process a constant stream of information and adjust their strategies in real time (Green & Bavelier, 2012).

Consider, for example, the fast-paced environment of a strategy game. Players must assess the status of their resources, the actions of opponents, and the changing dynamics of the battlefield. This continuous assessment fosters decision-making skills, as each choice can have significant consequences on the game's outcome. It prompts players to practice weighing potential risks and benefits quickly, often leading to improved decision-making skills in real-world contexts (Przybylski, 2014).

Similarly, video games that involve time pressure and quick reflexes can significantly boost processing speed. Many games require players to make split-second decisions, react to stimuli, and execute complex actions swiftly. Research indicates that regular engagement with such games can lead to faster information processing and improved attention to detail in everyday life (Dye et al., 2009).

Moreover, adaptability, or cognitive flexibility, is another executive function that benefits from video gameplay. Games often present players with novel scenarios that require quick shifts in tactics. This is especially true in sandbox games, where players are given the freedom to explore and engage with dynamic environments. The brain, when exposed to these changing contexts, learns to adapt by forming and strengthening neural connections, which in turn enhances overall cognitive flexibility (Boot et al., 2008).

A notable example of a game that promotes adaptability is Minecraft. Its open-world design and player-driven interactions necessitate continuous adaptation to new challenges. Players learn to modify their strategies as they encounter different biomes, resources, and threats. This kind of gameplay encourages creative problem-solving and the ability to adjust one's approach—a skill that's essential not just in gaming, but in life.

Importantly, certain games can also foster emotional regulation, a crucial component of executive function. Engaging in cooperative or role-playing games, for instance, may enhance emotional intelligence by requiring players to interpret non-verbal cues and manage interpersonal dynamics (Granic et al., 2014). This aspect of gaming can augment a child's ability to navigate social environments, fostering empathy and improved emotional management.

Parents and educators might wonder how these findings translate into actionable advice. First and foremost, selecting games that are not only age-appropriate but also intricate enough to challenge executive functions is crucial. Games with strategic depth, diverse scenarios, and interactive complexity should be prioritized over simplistic or repetitive ones. It's also beneficial to incorporate discussions about gameplay into routine interactions, allowing children to reflect on their decision-making processes and strategic adjustments.

While the cognitive benefits of certain types of gaming are becoming clearer, it's vital to maintain a balanced perspective. Not all games are created equal, and excessive gaming can lead to negative outcomes such as impaired social skills, reduced physical activity, and overreliance on digital entertainment (Gentile et al., 2011). Therefore, setting healthy boundaries and encouraging activities that promote physical, cognitive, and emotional well-being alongside gaming is essential.

Additionally, involving children in a variety of experiences, including outdoor play and creative arts, can further bolster the cognitive skills enhanced by video games. This holistic approach ensures that the development of executive functions isn't isolated to a single domain. Instead, it integrates the benefits of gaming with broader educational and recreational practices.

In conclusion, while video games have often been scrutinized for potential negative impacts, a growing body of research highlights their potential benefits for enhancing executive functions such as decision-making, processing speed, and adaptability. By selecting appropriate games and maintaining a balanced lifestyle, caregivers can empower children to harness these benefits, supporting their cognitive and emotional development in meaningful and impactful ways.

Strategy & Problem-Solving Skills in Interactive Games

Interactive games are not just a source of entertainment for children; they have the potential to function as tools for brain development, particularly in enhancing strategy and problem-solving skills. As our digital landscape expands, it becomes increasingly important for parents and caregivers to recognize how these games can contribute to a child's cognitive growth. While there's a myriad of games available, strategic games stand out for their ability to engage children in complex decision-making processes in a fun and engaging manner.

Unlike passive activities, interactive games require players to continually assess their environment, consider possible outcomes, and make decisions that will influence the game's progression. This dynamic engagement promotes critical thinking and problem-solving abilities, which are essential skills in both academic and real-world settings. For instance, games that involve building structures or managing resources teach kids the value of planning and foresight, helping them develop an understanding of cause and effect (Granic et al., 2014).

Strategy in games often involves identifying patterns, predicting opponents' moves, and adapting strategies swiftly. These experiences can be particularly beneficial for children as they mirror many complex cognitive processes happening in other areas of life and learning. By learning to adjust their tactics based on new information or changing environments, kids develop their cognitive flexibility, which is crucial for adaptability in an ever-changing world (Bavelier et al., 2012).

Furthermore, problem-solving within games often requires players to work through a series of challenges or puzzles to advance to the next level. This kind of iterative thinking encourages perseverance and resilience as children learn to analyze situations, test hypotheses, and refine their approaches to reach solutions. Success in these games often relies on a willingness to experiment and learn from mistakes, which can foster a growth mindset and a love for learning (Dweck, 2006).

In addition to individual challenges, many interactive games include collaborative elements where players must communicate and strategize with others to achieve common goals. This cooperative gameplay can enhance social skills and emotional intelligence by encouraging teamwork, communication, and empathy. Children learn to appreciate different perspectives and develop negotiation skills, which are invaluable in both personal and professional relationships.

However, it's important for parents and educators to be selective about the games children are exposed to, ensuring they are age-appropriate and offer constructive challenges without overwhelming young minds. It's also crucial to balance gaming with other activities that promote overall well-being, such as physical exercise and face-to-face interactions, to ensure that children receive a holistic approach to cognitive and emotional development (Anderson et al., 2010).

To optimize the potential benefits of strategic and problem-solving games, parents and caregivers should consider setting boundaries on gaming time while emphasizing the quality of content. It is possible to cultivate an environment where digital play becomes a supplement to traditional learning and growth, aiding in the development of essential life skills. Carefully selected interactive games, when used conscientiously, can be effective tools in enhancing the strategic and problem-solving skills that are foundational to a child's future success.

Together, parents, educators, and game developers can collaborate to create a digital environment where interactive play is a catalyst for cognitive advancement rather than a detriment. By focusing on games that require thoughtful strategy and adaptive problem-solving, we can help children foster the skills necessary to navigate a complex and ever-evolving world with confidence and competence. As with many tools available to us in child development, moderation and mindful application hold the keys to unlocking potential.

Enhancing Memory & Cognitive Flexibility Through Digital Play

In a world increasingly driven by digital interactions, understanding the potential cognitive benefits of video games and digital play has become crucial for parents and educators. Contrary to the earlier belief that video games solely foster negative effects on children's behavior and development, recent research highlights that these digital tools can enhance memory and cognitive flexibility (Granic et al., 2014).

Cognitive flexibility, a component of executive functions, refers to the brain's ability to adapt to new situations, change perspectives, and manage competing tasks. Video games often require players to switch between multiple goals, rules, and tasks rapidly, cultivating this flexibility. For instance, strategy games, where players must anticipate opponents' moves or adapt strategy based on evolving scenarios, give the brain a workout equivalent to learning how to navigate complex social situations (Bavelier & Green, 2019).

Memory enhancement through video games is another significant area of interest for researchers. Games often involve complex worlds, intricate storylines, and numerous tasks, which can lead to improvements in working memory. Working memory is crucial for learning and reasoning, and it's directly engaged when players plan actions, follow storylines, and remember past information relevant to future decisions. Through this engaged interaction, video games can serve as practical exercises for the brain to process and retain information effectively (Kühn et al., 2014).

Importantly, not all games are created equal in their cognitive benefits. Educational games, designed with specific learning outcomes in mind, can particularly enhance cognitive skills by providing players with challenges that are both entertaining and educational. For example, brain-training games that use puzzles and problem-solving tasks specifically target and improve various aspects of cognitive functioning.

These games can stimulate neural pathways associated with memory, attention, and logical reasoning, often revealing improvements after consistent use.

A well-designed digital play environment can mimic the complexities of real-world problem-solving scenarios. This effect is evident in role-playing games (RPGs), where participants must manage resources, strategize, and interact with other virtual characters. These activities can foster decision-making skills and adaptive thinking, as they require players to respond to the game's feedback and modify their strategies accordingly. As a result, gamers often develop a knack for creative problem-solving and critical thinking, skills that are highly valuable in everyday life (Przybylski & Mishra, 2016).

Moreover, some games integrate elements of social interaction, encouraging teamwork and collaborative problem-solving. Online multiplayer games provide opportunities for users to work together toward common goals, communicate effectively, and develop negotiation skills. These social aspects of gaming can enhance emotional intelligence and empathy, as players learn to recognize and respond to the emotions and actions of others within the game environment. This kind of cooperative gameplay can also translate to real-life interpersonal settings, facilitating better emotional understanding and communication skills (Kaye et al., 2017).

While these potential benefits present an optimistic picture of digital play, it's crucial to approach digital playtime with intention and monitoring. Overindulgence or lack of a structured gaming environment can lead to negative outcomes, such as unhealthy screen time habits and cognitive overload. Balancing gaming with other activities and maintaining productive digital use remains key. Parents and educators should guide children in choosing games that offer educational value and foster beneficial cognitive skills while setting limits consistent with healthy lifestyle practices.

As we navigate the impact of video games and digital play on brain development, awareness and knowledge are powerful tools. By strategically selecting and regulating the kinds of games children engage with, adults can harness the compelling nature of digital play to serve educational and developmental purposes. This approach not only safeguards against harmful effects but also enriches a child's cognitive toolkit, preparing them to excel in an increasingly complex world.

With intentional use and careful selection, digital play can indeed be a valuable ally in promoting memory and cognitive development. By fostering a balanced approach that combines digital adventures with traditional learning activities, we give children a well-rounded cognitive environment where their potential can thrive.

Educational & Brain-Training Games: Do They Really Work?

We live in an age where the allure of technology and its promises draw us into new territories of learning and engagement. Parents and educators alike are keenly interested in understanding whether educational and brain-training games are truly effective in enhancing cognitive abilities in children or if they're merely clever marketing ploys. Although the answer isn't straightforward, exploring the nature of these games and their impact on brain development provides valuable insights.

Emerging research indicates that some educational and brain-training games can indeed offer cognitive benefits. These games often emphasize skills such as memory, attention, and problem-solving, aspects of cognition that are pivotal for academic success and daily functioning (Bavelier et al., 2012). For example, certain games require players to identify patterns, manage tasks under time constraints, or solve puzzles, all of which can help to sharpen various cognitive processes. Brain-training games often claim to target and strengthen specific brain areas that might otherwise remain underdeveloped, leading to better overall cognitive function.

However, it's crucial to differentiate between different types of games. Not every digital game branded as "educational" provides substantial cognitive benefits. Many games labeled for educational purposes might only offer a superficial form of engagement. These games can sometimes be akin to digital worksheets, lacking interactive elements that encourage deep cognitive processing. Studies have shown that the best outcomes often come from games that incorporate adaptive difficulty levels, ensuring that challenges remain both attainable and stimulating for the user (Green & Bavelier, 2012).

Moreover, the context in which these games are played influences their effectiveness. The presence of parents or educators who can guide and contextualize the in-game learning experiences significantly enhances the impact of these games. When adults help children reflect on what they've learned or challenge them to apply new strategies, the cognitive benefits of these games can extend far beyond the screen (Gee, 2003).

While the short-term benefits of educational games are promising, long-term benefits are still under investigation. A critical question remains whether these digital skills translate into improved real-world abilities. Some research suggests that the skills honed in these games, such as spatial awareness and strategic thinking, can indeed transfer to non-digital contexts, resulting in academic improvements in subjects like mathematics and science (Granic et al., 2014). However, more longitudinal studies are needed to fully understand the lasting impact of these educational tools.

The emotional and social aspects of gaming also deserve consideration. Structured educational games can foster a sense of accomplishment and resilience as children navigate and overcome in-game challenges. The positive reinforcement and feedback offered by these games may bolster a child's self-confidence and motivation to tackle other learning tasks. Furthermore, multi-player games promote collaboration and communication skills, encouraging children to negotiate, share, and develop leadership abilities—all vital components of socio-emotional development (Gee, 2003).

Nonetheless, it's imperative to acknowledge the potential downsides of heavy reliance on brain-training games. Excessive screen time can lead to issues such as eye strain, reduced physical activity, and disrupted sleep patterns—all of which negatively impact a child's overall well-being (Cain & Gradisar, 2010). Additionally, while some games can be cognitively enriching, there's a risk of children becoming overly dependent on digital solutions for problem-solving, potentially reducing their creative and critical thinking capabilities when faced with real-world challenges.

Taking these factors into account, it becomes evident that educational and brain-training games can be a useful tool in a broader cognitive development strategy, but they shouldn't be the sole method. There needs to be a balanced approach where digital games complement traditional learning methods and other forms of cognitive engagement, like reading, physical activities, and interactive play. Looking beyond the screen, encouraging children to engage in a variety of mental and physical activities can lead to a more rounded developmental experience.

In summary, educational and brain-training games do hold the potential to boost cognitive and emotional growth, provided they are used thoughtfully and as part of a diverse toolkit. Parents, educators, and caregivers should look beyond the label and critically assess the content and nature of these games. Active involvement and guidance will not only enhance the learning experience but also ensure that children are reaping the full spectrum of benefits these games offer, preparing them for success both in school and in life.

Can Video Games Support Emotional Resilience & Stress Relief?

There's no denying that video games have become an integral part of many children's lives. While some adults may be skeptical of their benefits, research suggests that video games can promote emotional resilience and serve as a valuable tool for stress relief. Let's explore how these digital experiences might contribute positively to children's emotional well-being.

First and foremost, video games offer an escape from everyday stressors, providing children with a safe space to express themselves freely and experiment with different roles. This interactive form of engagement allows kids to disconnect from their immediate environment, giving their minds an opportunity to regroup and recharge. This temporary escape can be compared to losing oneself in a good book or becoming absorbed in a favorite hobby—activities that offer similar mental reprieve (Granic et al., 2014).

Moreover, many video games encourage social interaction through multiplayer modes, where players are either collaborating or competing. These interactions can foster a sense of community and belonging, important factors in building emotional resilience. For some children, especially those who struggle with face-to-face social interaction, online gaming can serve as a platform to build social skills and forge meaningful friendships (Cole & Griffiths, 2007). These online connections can provide emotional support and encouragement, further enhancing their ability to cope with everyday challenges.

Fostering emotional resilience also involves navigating failure and learning how to manage emotions in the face of defeat. Video games regularly present challenges that require players to try, fail, and try again. This cycle teaches kids perseverance and the notion that failure is a part of learning and growth. By experiencing setbacks in a controlled, low-stakes setting, children learn to handle disappointment and setbacks in real life more effectively. The quick feedback loop inherent in gaming helps them develop a mindset where resilience becomes a natural response to challenges (Dweck, 2006).

The immersive nature of video games often places players in high-stakes situations that require quick thinking and adaptive problem-solving. These scenarios can help reduce anxiety by engaging the player's focus, pulling their attention away from stressful thoughts and emotions. The sense of achievement felt after overcoming a difficult level or mastering a complex game can provide a significant boost to a child's self-esteem, an important component of emotional resilience (Przybylski & Weinstein, 2019).

Interestingly, certain types of games, particularly those with narrative elements, can enhance empathy and emotional understanding in players. Story-driven games often place players in the shoes of characters, requiring them to make decisions based on different perspectives. This experience of walking in someone else's shoes can promote empathy, a crucial skill in emotional intelligence and resilience (Bormann & Greitemeyer, 2015). The lessons learned from these virtual narratives can translate into real-world skills for understanding and relating to others on an emotional level.

In terms of stress relief, video games can serve as both a distraction and a form of active engagement. For instance, casual games designed for relaxation, such as those involving puzzles or creative tasks, can help calm the mind and reduce tension. These games often feature soothing music and graphics, contributing to a tranquil gaming environment. On the other hand, more action-oriented games might offer a healthy way to channel stress and frustration, giving players an outlet for energy and emotion that might otherwise build up unhealthily.

However, it is crucial to strike a balance, as excessive gaming can lead to negative outcomes such as sleep disturbances and social withdrawal. The key lies in moderating playtime and ensuring that gaming is part of a diverse range of activities that include exercise, outdoor play, and enough sleep. Additionally, parents and caregivers should pay attention to the content of games. Choosing age-appropriate games that promote positive values can enhance the constructive benefits of gaming experiences. Setting reasonable limits on gaming time and facilitating discussions about the content can help ensure that gaming remains a positive force in a child's development (Gentile et al., 2011).

While video games can support emotional resilience and stress relief, they should not replace traditional methods of stress management and emotional support. Encouraging practices such as mindfulness, regular physical activity, and open communication within the family are vital components of maintaining a well-rounded approach to emotional and psychological well-being. Ultimately, video games should complement these practices rather than serve as a standalone solution.

By understanding and leveraging the potential positive impacts of video games, parents and caregivers can ensure that digital play serves as a constructive part of a child's emotional development toolkit. When approached mindfully, video games can help children develop important life skills such as problem-solving, socialization, and emotional regulation, all of which are essential for navigating the complexities of modern life.

In integrating video games into children's lives, the most important factor remains thoughtful engagement. By actively participating in discussions about gaming content and establishing clear boundaries, caregivers can support and monitor their child's gaming habits effectively. This informed oversight helps in transforming video games from a potential source of concern into a valuable ally in fostering emotional resilience and stress relief.

The Risks & Downsides of Excessive Gaming

The vibrant world of digital gaming offers children and teenagers incredible opportunities to engage their minds, but excessive gaming can present significant risks and downsides. While some video games can enhance cognitive skills such as strategic thinking and problem-solving, these benefits can quickly be overshadowed by negative outcomes when gaming habits become excessive or addictive. This section delves into those potential downsides, offering insights for parents, teachers, and caregivers who aim to foster a balanced approach to digital play.

One of the most immediate concerns of excessive gaming is its impact on sleep. Video games often stimulate the brain with bright screens, rapid movement, and engaging narratives, potentially disrupting natural sleep patterns. When children and teenagers stay up late gaming, their sleep is often compromised, affecting their cognitive functions like memory, attention, and learning the following day. Studies have shown that poor sleep can lead to decreased academic performance and mood disturbances in children and adolescents (Fobian et al., 2016).

Moreover, excessive gaming often leads to sedentary behavior, which poses health risks in the short and long term. Children who spend long periods sitting and playing video games miss out on crucial physical activities that promote cardiovascular health, muscle development, and overall well-being. The allure of digital play might cause them to shun outdoor activities, which are vital for physical and mental development. Emerging research indicates that extended sedentary behavior in young people is associated with conditions such as obesity, metabolic syndrome, and decreased mental health outcomes (Tremblay et al., 2011).

The immersive nature of video games can sometimes be an escape from real-world responsibilities and interactions, leading to social isolation. While some games offer online social interaction, they don't fully replace face-to-face communication's depth and emotional benefits. Excessive gamers may develop a preference for virtual interactions over real-world socialization, potentially affecting their ability to build empathy, communicate effectively, and form meaningful relationships. Long-term social isolation can lead to emotional challenges such as loneliness and anxiety (Gentile et al., 2012).

Furthermore, the fast-paced and rewarding nature of many games can contribute to attention issues. Frequent exposure to rapid game environments can condition gamers to favor quick rewards and constant stimulation, potentially impairing their ability to sustain attention during less engaging real-world tasks like schoolwork. This can be particularly concerning for children with Attention Deficit Hyperactivity Disorder (ADHD) who already face challenges with sustained attention and impulse control.

Dopamine, a neurotransmitter associated with pleasure and reward, plays a significant role in gaming's addictive potential. Games are designed to provide immediate rewards, triggering dopamine release and reinforcing gaming behaviors. Over time, this can lead to a desensitization effect, where the gamer needs more gaming to achieve the same level of satisfaction. Such over-indulgence can create an addictive cycle, affecting focus, motivation, and emotional regulation (Weinstein, 2010).

Another noteworthy concern is how excessive gaming can contribute to conflict within the family. When gaming becomes a priority over responsibilities and family time, disputes can arise. Parents might struggle to set boundaries on screen time, and children might resist, leading to a stressful family environment. Establishing clear guidelines and encouraging open communication about gaming habits can mitigate these issues and promote a healthier balance.

The types of games children play can also influence the negative or positive outcomes of gaming. Not all games are created equal, and those saturated with violent or inappropriate content can impact children's behavior and emotional well-being. Although the link between violence in video games and aggressive behavior is still debated among researchers, exposure to violent content can desensitize children to violence and lead to more hostile behaviors (Anderson & Dill, 2000).

Lastly, it is crucial to consider how excessive gaming can interfere with personal development milestones. Time spent on gaming could otherwise be used for hobbies, academic work, or family activities. These alternative engagements are necessary for developing diverse skills, creativity, and a strong sense of identity. Finding a healthy balance between gaming and other activities is key to ensuring that children have rich and varied experiences that contribute to their growth and development.

In summary, excessive gaming presents several risks that can negatively affect brain development and overall well-being. While video games are not inherently harmful, the balance lies in moderation and mindfulness. Parents, teachers, and caregivers must foster environments that encourage varied, enriching activities alongside digital play. By setting boundaries and selecting appropriate content, adults can help children enjoy the benefits of gaming without falling into its potential pitfalls.

How Gaming Affects Sleep & the Brain's Recovery Cycle

The digital landscape has become an undeniable part of our children's lives, with video games occupying a notably significant portion of leisure time across many age groups. However, as these games continue to offer benefits such as problem-solving skills and cognitive flexibility, it is crucial to examine their impact on other aspects of well-being, particularly sleep. The relationship between gaming and sleep is complex and calls for an understanding that parents, teachers, and caregivers can apply in supporting healthy brain development.

While it's undeniable that certain video games can boost cognitive functions, playing them too close to bedtime can upset sleep patterns. Various studies indicate that exposure to the blue light emitted by screens can suppress melatonin production, a hormone that regulates sleep cycles, making it difficult for kids to fall asleep (Cajochen et al., 2011). In today's fast-paced world, where kids are constantly juggling learning, play, and social interactions, good sleep isn't just beneficial; it's essential. A poor night's sleep doesn't just result in a groggy morning—it impacts the brain's ability to recover and rejuvenate, affecting mood, attention, and memory regulation (Carskadon, 2011).

Disrupted sleep doesn't just bring short-term consequences. Consistently inadequate rest can negatively affect a child's learning abilities. When children stay up late gaming, they often enter stages of sleep deprivation that hinder memory consolidation—an essential process for learning new information (Stickgold, 2005). This can lead to challenges in school and social settings, where retaining and applying new information is key. A child who is cognitively fatigued will struggle to reach their full potential both academically and emotionally.

It's not just the length of sleep that video gaming can disrupt but also its quality. Sleep is a cycle, comprising varying stages that each serve pivotal roles in overall health. The rapid eye movement (REM) stage, linked to dreaming, is especially crucial for cognitive restoration. Engaging in digital play before bed can interrupt these crucial stages; games often require a heightened state of alertness and increased emotional involvement, delaying the onset of deep sleep cycles (Higuchi et al., 2005). As a result, even if a child gets a full nine hours of sleep, they may still wake up feeling unrested.

Parents and caregivers must equip themselves with realistic strategies to ensure that gaming, although inherently engaging, doesn't hinder sleep. Setting screen-time boundaries, such as banning screens an hour before bed, can let natural melatonin levels return to normal. Encouraging activities that promote relaxation before sleep—like reading or mild stretching—can also be effective.

In conjunction with setting firm boundaries, it's beneficial to develop a structured bedtime routine. A consistent routine signals the brain and body that it's time to wind down and prepares them for rest. This alignment isn't just beneficial in curbing gaming tendencies; it's a holistic approach that nurtures all aspects of brain health.

A part of helping children transition away from evening gaming and towards healthier routines involves education. Explain the brain's need for sleep and the effects of gaming on its recovery processes in terms they can understand. Rather than banning video games outright, facilitating a balanced approach where children learn self-regulation can be immensely beneficial. They gain autonomy and a sense of responsibility for their overall health.

Finally, while exploring the connection between gaming and sleep, it is necessary to consider the individual differences among children. Some might be more affected by gaming than others. Therefore, observe and adapt—watch the child's mood, academic performance, and energy levels. Tailoring the approach to meet each child's unique needs offers the best chance for success.

By understanding the intricate dance between gaming, sleep, and the brain's recovery cycle, caregivers can make informed decisions about children's digital engagement. The aim shouldn't be to eliminate gaming but to integrate it in a way that supports not just cognitive and emotional growth but the overall developmental trajectory. With the right strategies, gaming can be part of a healthy lifestyle that fosters a vibrant, well-rested mind.

Dopamine Overload & Video Game Addiction: How It Impacts Focus & Motivation

In today's digital age, video games have become a ubiquitous part of many children's lives, offering immersive experiences that captivate and engage. Yet, as compelling as these games are, they also pose significant challenges, particularly concerning dopamine overload and addiction. Dopamine, a neurotransmitter involved in reward and pleasure pathways in the brain, plays a crucial role in motivation and focus. But what happens when this natural system is overstimulated by excessive gaming? Understanding this process is essential for parents, educators, and caregivers aiming to foster healthy cognitive and emotional development in children.

The immediate appeal of video games lies predominantly in their ability to trigger the brain's reward system. Each achievement or level completed in a game results in a burst of dopamine, reinforcing the behavior and making players crave more gaming time. While occasional gaming can have cognitive benefits, such as improved coordination and problem-solving skills, overindulgence can hijack the brain's reward circuits, leading to reduced motivation for other activities like homework, outdoor play, or social interactions (Bailey, 2021).

As the brain is constantly seeking the next dopamine fix from gaming, the ability to maintain interest and concentration on less stimulating, yet equally important tasks wanes. This phenomenon isn't exclusive to gaming; however, video games tend to be particularly potent due to their fast-paced, interactive nature. The anticipation of the next reward in a game can surpass that of traditional learning tasks, making it hard for educators to compete with the allure of digital play (Greenfield & DeWinstanley, 2020).

The implications of this dopamine-driven behavior are substantial. The National Institute of Mental Health highlights that heightened exposure to digital screens and gaming can result in attention deficits, reduced impulse control, and lack of motivation in school-aged children (NIMH, 2022). These children might find it challenging to focus on lengthy or monotonous tasks, leading to lower academic performance and engagement.

Parents and caregivers may notice that their child shows remarkable persistence and focus during gaming, but struggles to bring the same dedication to homework or household chores. This discrepancy is often due to the lack of immediate rewards or dopamine boosts that everyday tasks offer compared to video games. It's a dilemma that requires strategic intervention and balanced management of screen time.

One effective approach to counteracting the effects of dopamine overload is promoting alternative activities that naturally engage the brain's motivation and pleasure pathways. Physical exercise, for instance, is known to release endorphins and serotonin, chemicals that also contribute to feelings of reward and satisfaction. Encouraging regular breaks for outdoor play or participation in team sports can help reset the brain's reward thresholds and improve overall well-being (Ratey & Hagerman, 2008).

Moreover, fostering intrinsic motivation is crucial. Unlike extrinsic rewards that video games provide, intrinsic motivation comes from finding joy and satisfaction in the activity itself. Encouraging children to pursue interests that captivate them without the need for digital reinforcement can rebuild their ability to focus over longer stretches. This could be cultivating hobbies like art, music, or crafting, which offer a tangible sense of progress and achievement.

Establishing clear boundaries around gaming time and emphasizing digital play as a privilege rather than a right can also help manage expectations. Setting time limits and ensuring that gaming doesn't encroach on academic responsibilities or family time is vital. Furthermore, discussing the reasons behind these limits with children helps them understand the importance of a balanced lifestyle and reduces resistance to boundaries (Anderson et al., 2017).

It's equally important to adopt a collaborative approach with educators and healthcare providers. Teachers can integrate elements of gamification in classroom settings to capture students' interests in education-based tasks, thus reinforcing schoolwork as rewarding and significant. For children demonstrating signs of gaming addiction, consulting a child psychologist or a behavioral therapist can provide valuable insight and strategies to manage digital habits.

As we navigate this digital landscape, understanding the balance between digital entertainment and holistic development will remain imperative. After all, while video games serve as a modern playground for creativity and strategy, they should complement rather than overshadow the myriad of learning experiences that foster a well-rounded and healthy brain development process for our children.

In conclusion, by recognizing the signs of dopamine overload and strategically guiding children's interactions with video games, we can safeguard their focus and motivation. We can empower them to engage more fully with the world around them—not just the digital one—and equip them with the mental tools needed for success in various facets of life.

Increased Sedentary Behavior & the Health Risks of a Digital-Only Lifestyle

As we navigate the digital age, it's clear that technology has become deeply integrated into the daily lives of children and adolescents. While this integration has its benefits, such as access to information and educational tools, it also brings with it the challenge of increased sedentary behavior. This shift towards a more sedentary lifestyle has profound implications for children's health, including both physical and cognitive aspects.

The term "sedentary behavior" primarily refers to activities that involve low energy expenditure, such as sitting or lying down while engaging in activities like watching screens or playing video games. The proliferation of digital devices and their seemingly ubiquitous presence in children's lives have led to reduced physical activity levels. With children spending more time glued to screens, they face a host of health risks that parents, teachers, and caregivers must address.

One of the most immediate concerns associated with a sedentary lifestyle is the risk of developing obesity. Studies have shown a strong correlation between high screen time and an increased risk of obesity in children (Tremblay et al., 2011). This risk stems from both the time spent inactive and the accompanying dietary habits, such as snacking on high-calorie, low-nutrition foods while engaged in screen time. Obesity can lead to numerous health complications, including diabetes, cardiovascular diseases, and joint issues, all of which can have long-term consequences if not addressed early.

Beyond physical health, increased sedentary behavior also impacts mental well-being. Research has indicated that excessive screen time can lead to issues such as depression and anxiety in young people (Twenge & Campbell, 2018). The underlying mechanisms are varied but may include factors like decreased physical activity, disruption of sleep patterns, and reduced opportunities for face-to-face social interactions. As children spend more time in front of screens, they miss out on valuable social experiences that are critical for emotional regulation and developing interpersonal skills.

Sleep disruption is another significant risk associated with excessive digital engagement. Many children use devices late into the night, exposing themselves to blue light emitted by screens, which can interfere with the body's natural circadian rhythms (Hale & Guan, 2015). This disruption can lead to inadequate or poor-quality sleep, which is vital for cognitive development, memory consolidation, and emotional stability. Furthermore, lack of sleep can exacerbate attention problems and contribute to behavioral issues, making it difficult for children to thrive academically and socially.

The cognitive impact of increased sedentary behavior also warrants attention. Studies have shown that physical activity is crucial for brain health and cognitive development (Hillman et al., 2008). Active play and exercise promote better blood circulation and oxygenation to the brain, which in turn supports neural growth and plasticity. When children spend more time being sedentary, they miss out on these essential benefits, potentially hindering their cognitive development and academic performance.

Maintaining a balance between screen time and physical activity is vital for fostering healthy development in children. Experts recommend limiting recreational screen time to no more than one to two hours per day while ensuring that children engage in at least one hour of moderate to vigorous physical activity each day (American Academy of Pediatrics, 2016). This balance encourages children to cultivate healthy habits that include physical exercise, outdoor play, and structured activities that stimulate both their bodies and minds.

Parents and caregivers play a crucial role in modeling and promoting active lifestyles. Encouraging activities such as family walks, bike rides, or outdoor sports can help reduce the amount of time children spend on sedentary activities. Schools also have a critical role in integrating physical activity into the daily routine, providing opportunities for students to engage in sports and active play during recess and physical education classes.

Furthermore, it's essential to foster environments that support limited screen use and encourage balanced media consumption. Creating screen-free zones in the home, particularly in bedrooms and dining areas, can help establish boundaries and promote healthier habits. Setting clear expectations and guidelines around screen time, and promoting activities that encourage creativity and physical engagement, can guide children toward a more balanced lifestyle.

Digital-only lifestyles may seem convenient and entertaining, but acknowledging and addressing the associated health risks is vital. By actively reducing sedentary behavior and encouraging more dynamic forms of play and interaction, parents, teachers, and caregivers can support children's physical health, cognitive development, and overall well-being. By doing so, we provide children with the tools they need to thrive both in the digital world and beyond.

Social Isolation vs. Social Gaming: When Is It Harmful?

The line between social connectivity and isolation in the realm of video gaming is thin and often complex. Video games can offer a unique digital playground that connects players with peers across the globe, fostering a sense of community and shared experience. However, they also have the potential to entrap children and teens in a cycle of social withdrawal, blurring the lines between healthy interaction and harmful isolation. So, when do these digital interactions become detrimental to a child's development, and what can caregivers do to maintain a healthy balance?

First, it's essential to recognize that not all gaming is inherently harmful. Many video games are designed to be social experiences. Multiplayer online games, for example, can cultivate teamwork, communication, and problem-solving skills in ways that are both engaging and educational (Granic et al., 2014). Such games often involve players working together to achieve common goals, leading to a sense of camaraderie and belonging. For children who may feel marginalized in traditional social settings, this can be incredibly empowering and offer a renewed sense of identity.

However, problems arise when gaming becomes a solitary activity that replaces face-to-face interactions. Prolonged periods spent in isolation while gaming can lead to a reduction in social interactions, potentially impacting a child's social skills and emotional well-being. According to research, excessive gaming can contribute to social anxiety and withdrawal, manifesting in reduced participation in real-world activities (Lemmens et al., 2015). When a child opts for a virtual world over real-world interactions consistently, it should signal caregivers to step in and assess the dynamics at play.

Understanding why some children retreat into gaming is crucial. Often, children who feel misunderstood or lack self-esteem might find solace in the identities they can assume within games. Gaming allows for experimentation with different personas and the feeling of achievement without fear of judgment or failure. While these experiences can be positive, they may also become an unhealthy escape from reality, detaching the child from the physical world (Chiu et al., 2004). Striking the right balance is a nuanced task that requires empathy and attention from parents and caregivers.

Another vital factor to consider is the content of the games themselves. Not all social gaming is equal, and the impact of a game on a child's mental health is often related to its content. Cooperative strategy games, for instance, are known to improve cognitive functions and can even help in developing patience and strategic thinking. On the other hand, games that glorify violence or negative behaviors could potentially have adverse effects, including increasing aggression and desensitizing children to violence (Anderson et al., 2010). It's important for caregivers to be aware of what games their children are playing and the types of interactions these games encourage.

The challenge, therefore, is not to eliminate gaming but to create a balanced approach where digital play complements, rather than replaces, other social activities. Encourage children to participate in physical activities and outdoor play, which are vital for healthy growth. Set aside specific times for gaming, ensuring these are nestled between various offline interactions and responsibilities. This balanced approach can help children enjoy the benefits of social gaming without succumbing to the pitfalls of isolation.

Communication is key in this balance. Engage with children about their gaming experiences, showing genuine interest in the games they play. Discussing their reasons for gaming and their feelings about it encourages open dialogue and provides insights into their online world. It also helps in guiding them towards making choices that support both their social and cognitive development.

Incorporating these strategies can foster an environment where children can enjoy the positive aspects of digital social gaming while mitigating risks of social isolation. Knowing when gaming habits are crossing into unhealthy territory can sometimes be challenging, but by being observant and proactive, caregivers can take steps to ensure a healthy digital balance for their children. It's about guiding them to navigate both the digital and physical worlds with confidence and balance.

Ultimately, while video games offer avenues for social interaction and cognitive benefits, the potential for isolation is a reality that shouldn't be ignored. Caregivers play a crucial role in ensuring that gaming acts as a bridge to more comprehensive social experiences, rather than a barrier. By fostering healthy gaming habits and maintaining open communication, caregivers can help children develop into well-rounded individuals who can flourish in both the digital and real worlds.

The Link Between Fast-Paced Gaming & Attention Issues

As digital landscapes evolve, fast-paced video games captivate millions of children and teenagers across the globe. These games often demand rapid reactions, quick decision-making, and an intense focus over prolonged periods. While they can offer certain cognitive benefits, a growing body of research indicates a potential link between this style of gaming and attention-related issues in young players. The fast-action nature of these games could impact a child's ability to focus and sustain attention on non-gaming activities, potentially interfering with their cognitive and emotional development.

Studies have shown that fast-paced video games can influence the brain's attention systems by overloading them. When constantly engaging in rapid, high-stimulus gaming, children's brains may become conditioned to expect and require high levels of stimulation to sustain attention. This expectation can make everyday tasks, like homework or participating in classroom activities, feel unstimulating in comparison, leading to shorter attention spans and increased distractibility (Gentile et al., 2012).

The design of these games is often tied to immediate rewards or penalties, a mechanism that can foster a pattern of instant gratification. As children repeatedly experience these quick reward cycles, they may develop a reliance on immediate feedback, making them less patient with tasks that require longer-term effort and focus. This propensity can hinder a child's ability to persevere with challenging tasks, a critical skill underpinning both academic and real-world success (Kardefelt-Winther, 2017).

A significant factor in the attention-related issues arising from fast-paced gaming is its impact on the brain's dopamine pathways. Dopamine, a neurotransmitter, plays an essential role in motivating behavior and directing attention. When engaged in gaming, especially those designed to be fast-paced, children's brains can experience an overproduction of dopamine, leading to an "overloaded" reward system. This alteration may contribute to difficulties in sustaining attention on less stimulating activities and even lead to symptoms similar to Attention Deficit Hyperactivity Disorder (ADHD) (Zheng et al., 2019).

It is important to approach the conversation about gaming and attention issues with nuance and understanding. While some children might exhibit signs of attention difficulties linked to their gaming habits, others might not experience any adverse effects. Individual differences, such as a child's baseline attentional control, parental involvement, and the type of games played, all play critical roles in determining the potential impact on attention. Researchers recommend a balanced engagement with digital media while ensuring that children have ample opportunities for various forms of play and activities that promote sustained attention and self-regulation (Gentile et al., 2012).

For parents and caregivers, setting boundaries and establishing healthy gaming habits is crucial. Start by promoting a variety of activities that engage different attention and cognitive systems, such as reading, outdoor play, and structured sports. These activities can aid in balancing the fast-paced nature of video games by providing experiences that support attention development in different contexts. Encouraging regular breaks during gaming sessions and sticking to recommended screen time limits are fundamental strategies that can help mitigate the negative impacts of fast-paced gaming (Kardefelt-Winther, 2017).

Furthermore, discussing the nature of gaming content with children can instill an awareness of its impacts on attention and behavior. Parents and educators can encourage kids to reflect on how they feel before, during, and after gaming sessions, promoting mindfulness about their digital consumption. This reflective exercise can help children become more attuned to their attention capabilities and learning patterns.

The research suggests that mindfulness practices, such as meditation and deep breathing, might also counteract some of the overstimulating effects of fast-paced gaming. These techniques can bolster a child's capacity for sustained attention by enhancing their ability to regulate emotional responses and focus on present-moment tasks. Encouraging mindfulness activities can serve as a valuable tool in helping children manage the fast-paced stimuli that come with gaming (Zheng et al., 2019).

Ultimately, while there is a clear potential link between fast-paced gaming and attention issues, it is only one piece of the complex puzzle of cognitive development. Parents, caregivers, and educators play a pivotal role in crafting a balanced digital environment for children. By fostering varied, enriching experiences outside of gaming and setting thoughtful boundaries around digital play, we can help support children's cognitive and emotional growth, ensuring that screen time remains a healthy part of their overall development.

Finding the Right Balance

In a world where digital entertainment is as immersive as ever, finding the right balance between video gaming and other activities becomes crucial for the well-being of children and teens. Video games have evolved from simple recreational tools to complex experiences that can enhance cognitive abilities but also present risks if indulged excessively. The challenge for parents, teachers, and caregivers lies in managing this dichotomy, ensuring that children reap the benefits without the adverse effects.

Over the years, research has shown that playing video games can offer varied cognitive benefits. Games that require strategic thinking, problem-solving, and quick decision-making can enhance executive function. These skills are pivotal for mental agility and adaptability, traits that serve children well in academic and real-life situations (Bavelier & Green, 2019). However, it's not just about choosing the right games—it's also about setting the right limits. Too much of anything can be harmful, and when it comes to digital play, moderation is key.

Setting boundaries around screen time is one crucial strategy. The American Academy of Pediatrics (AAP) recommends that children aged 6 and older have consistent limits on the time spent using media, ensuring it doesn't interfere with adequate sleep, physical activity, and other behaviors essential to health (AAP, 2016). It's also essential for families to create a media plan that considers each child's age, health, personality, and developmental stage. This approach helps tailor screen time rules that fit the unique needs of each child, fostering an environment where digital play is beneficial rather than detrimental.

Moreover, it's crucial to encourage a variety of activities outside of gaming. Physical exercise, social interactions, and creative play are all vital components of a balanced lifestyle that promote health and brain development. Outdoor play has been linked to improved mood and cognitive function, contributing to a well-rounded development (Roe & Aspinall, 2011). Encouraging children to engage in active play and spend time outdoors complements the cognitive benefits gained through digital games by providing physical exercise and opportunities for face-to-face socialization.

Choosing the right types of games is another component of finding balance. While fast-paced, adrenaline-fueled games can be exciting, they may also contribute to attention issues. Conversely, educational and strategy games, which require careful consideration and forethought, can reinforce patience and strategic thinking, aligning better with cognitive and emotional development goals. Thus, a discerning approach to selecting games that support cognitive health is imperative.

Another factor in balancing gaming habits is the role of parents and caregivers in modeling digital behaviors. Parents who demonstrate responsible screen use and prioritize offline interactions often see similar habits mirrored in their children. Creating tech-free times and spaces at home can encourage more mindful media consumption. For instance, designating times where screens are put away, like during meals or family events, can enhance family bonding and ensure more opportunities for face-to-face communication.

Equally important is addressing the common concerns about the potential negative impact of excessive gaming. Video game addiction, characterized by obsessive gaming behaviors and withdrawal symptoms when not playing, is increasingly recognized as a significant issue. Children who spend too much time gaming can suffer from disrupted sleep cycles, lower social engagement, and reduced academic performance (Gentile, 2009). Hence, recognizing the signs of gaming addiction is critical for timely intervention and support.

Finally, open communication between caregivers and children about gaming habits is essential. Discussing the games children play, what they find enjoyable, and what they might be learning from them can help adults guide children toward more beneficial gaming experiences. Regular conversations also allow parents to set expectations and boundaries collaboratively, ensuring children feel involved in the decision-making process and more likely to adhere to agreed-upon rules.

In conclusion, video games and digital play are not inherently harmful, but they do require thoughtful oversight to ensure they contribute positively to brain development. By understanding the potential benefits and risks, creating a balanced schedule that incorporates diverse activities, and maintaining open communication, caregivers can help children develop healthy gaming habits that enhance cognitive growth and emotional well-being.

Healthy Screen Time & Gaming Limits by Age Group

In the digital era, screens are an inescapable part of everyday life, impacting everything from education to entertainment. While they offer numerous benefits, like access to a wealth of information and opportunities for social interaction, they also pose challenges for children's brain development. The crux of this issue lies in establishing healthy screen time and gaming limits tailored to suit each age group's unique developmental needs.

For infants and toddlers, ages 0 to 2, the American Academy of Pediatrics (AAP) recommends avoiding screen time altogether, except for video chatting. At this critical stage of brain development, real-world interactions are far more valuable. The rapid growth of neural connections necessitates a sensory-rich environment filled with human touch, voice, and emotional responsiveness (AAP, 2016). Studies show that screen exposure at this age can hinder language acquisition and delay cognitive milestones (Zimmerman et al., 2007).

Preschoolers, ages 3 to 5, can benefit from limited screen interaction, but the content should be educational and interactive rather than passive. The AAP suggests no more than one hour per day, emphasizing co-viewing with adults to allow for discussions that enhance learning and understanding (AAP, 2016). High-quality programming that encourages cognitive engagement supports the development of essential skills such as language growth and problem-solving abilities.

As children enter elementary school, from ages 6 to 12, the focus shifts toward maintaining a balance between screen activities and other developmental pursuits like physical play, reading, and social interaction. While recreational screen time can extend to two hours a day, parents and caregivers need to closely monitor the content and context, ensuring it's age-appropriate and positively contributes to development. Non-screen activities such as outdoor play and exercise are critical for growth and emotional well-being, with screens ideally reserved for educational purposes or moderated gaming that fosters skills like strategic thinking and adaptability (Granic et al., 2014).

The teenage years, ages 13 to 18, present a distinctive set of challenges, especially as teenagers seek autonomy and are susceptible to peer influence. While technology can serve as a tool for education and social connection, excessive gaming and screen time can contribute to issues like poor sleep, reduced attention spans, and increased anxiety

(Twenge et al., 2018). Encouraging teenagers to participate in non-digital hobbies, sports, and face-to-face social activities is crucial in maintaining balance. Open dialogue about their digital experiences allows teenagers to partake in self-regulation of their habits, which is crucial for developing executive functioning skills.

Managing screen time effectively also involves fostering an environment where digital boundaries are respected. Establishing schedules that clearly delineate time for screens, chores, homework, and physical activity helps children and teens acclimate to diversified daily routines that prioritize overall well-being. Consistency and firm yet empathetic guidance from caregivers play integral roles in instilling these habits. Furthermore, modeling healthy screen habits as adults can significantly influence children's behavior.

Universal guidelines stress taking frequent breaks to alleviate screen fatigue, a practice beneficial for all age groups. The 20-20-20 rule—taking a 20-second break to look at something 20 feet away every 20 minutes of screen time—can help mitigate the physical toll on young eyes and enhance focus when re-engaging with digital content.

Part of setting these limits involves understanding the content accessed by children. Not all screen time is equal. While gaming can improve certain cognitive abilities like visual-spatial skills and decision-making, games that are excessively violent or addictive should be avoided. Educational games or those that encourage problem-solving and collaboration can be beneficial. Regular family discussions about content and its effects on mood and behavior can provide insights into how screen time impacts emotional health, serving as a cue for necessary adjustments.

It's essential for caregivers and educators to regularly evaluate each child's or teen's screen habits. These checks can identify shifts in mood, social behavior, or academic performance that may indicate unhealthy screen use. When necessary, working with professionals like pediatric psychologists or child development specialists can guide in establishing or adjusting technology-use strategies that support a child's cognitive and emotional growth.

In summary, while digital devices and gaming provide opportunities for learning and interaction, their impact on brain development heavily depends on how they're integrated into daily life. Establishing healthy screen time and gaming limits tailored to each age group, alongside non-digital activities, can optimize a child's cognitive and emotional development, ensuring that technology serves as a friend rather than a foe in nurturing a developing mind.

Choosing Games That Support Cognitive & Emotional Health

Selecting the right video games for kids isn't just about fun—it's an opportunity to bolster cognitive and emotional growth. Video games often get a bad rap, but when chosen wisely, they can serve as a valuable tool in a child's developmental journey. With a wide array of games designed to engage the brain, it's crucial for parents, teachers, and caregivers to identify those that enhance rather than hinder a child's development.

Firstly, it's essential to understand the game's content and its impact on the child. Educational games that focus on problem-solving, logical reasoning, and strategy can significantly benefit cognitive development. Games like "Minecraft," for instance, encourage creativity by allowing players to construct intricate structures while managing resources, promoting problem-solving skills in an engaging way.

Research supports the notion that certain video games can enhance cognitive capabilities, including processing speed, memory, and spatial reasoning. A study by Kühn et al. (2014) revealed that playing platform games like "Super Mario" can lead to structural brain changes associated with increased gray matter in regions responsible for navigation and strategic planning.

Interactive games that require multitasking and decision making can also train a child's executive functions. These games often demand that players make quick decisions based on rapidly changing visual and auditory stimuli, thereby sharpening attentional control and adaptability. Games such as "StarCraft II" are noted for their ability to improve cognitive flexibility and strategic thinking due to their complex, real-time strategic challenges (Basak, Boot, Voss, & Kramer, 2008).

Beyond cognitive benefits, certain games can also bolster emotional resilience and social skills. Multiplayer games can foster teamwork and communication, helping children to develop social bonds and learn to collaborate effectively. Games such as "Animal Crossing" and "Among Us" promote empathy, cooperation, and negotiation skills, offering a social platform that's respectful and inclusive.

However, it's crucial to monitor the content and ensure it aligns with your child's emotional maturity and cognitive capabilities. Games with violent or inappropriate themes may have adverse effects. Parents should carefully vet games and prioritize those that match the developmental stage of their child. The Entertainment Software Rating Board (ESRB) provides valuable ratings and descriptions that can guide these choices.

To maintain healthy gaming habits, it's beneficial to establish clear rules around gaming time. Consistent routines promote balance, preventing gaming from interfering with critical activities such as schoolwork, physical activities, and family time. The American Academy of Pediatrics recommends that screen time for children aged 6 and older should be consistent, curating a balance that supports both digital and physical play.

While the lure of excessive gaming time can be strong, combining digital play with physical activities is vital. Encourage games that incorporate physical movements, like those available on platforms such as the Nintendo Switch with "Just Dance" or the "Ring Fit Adventure", which encourage physical activity and engagement.

For educators and caregivers interested in integrating digital play into learning environments, it's worth exploring games that align with educational goals. Games that focus on STEM (Science, Technology, Engineering, and Mathematics) concepts, such as "Kerbal Space Program," can be highly effective. These games engage children in critical thinking and scientific inquiry, fostering an interest in science and technology fields (Steinkuehler & Duncan, 2008).

In conclusion, choosing games that support cognitive and emotional health requires mindful selection and active engagement in a child's digital life. By focusing on games that promote problem-solving, collaboration, and healthy social interaction, parents and caregivers can unlock the positive potential of digital play. As with most things, moderation and balance are key, ensuring that gaming enhances rather than detracts from overall development.

Understanding the benefits and risks associated with video games can empower caregivers to make informed choices. It's not just about setting limits but also about actively engaging with the child's digital experiences. Encouraging discussions about the games they're playing, exploring their interests, and being present during their gaming sessions can turn video games into an enriching part of a child's development journey.

Encouraging Outdoor Play & Physical Activity Alongside Digital Play

In today's digital age, where screens are omnipresent and technology influences nearly every aspect of life, the balance between digital and physical experiences becomes more critical than ever. As parents, teachers, and caregivers embrace the advantages of digital play, it's equally important to advocate for outdoor play and physical activity to ensure well-rounded development for children. The goal isn't to eliminate digital play but to harmonize it with physical experiences that nurture both body and mind.

Outdoor play provides children with opportunities to develop crucial motor skills, enhance their imagination, and improve their social interactions. When children climb, run, or play in natural settings, they engage in activities that bolster their physical health, coordination, and balance. Moreover, the sensory experience of being outdoors - the feel of the breeze, the scent of flowers, the sound of birds - contributes to a child's emotional and cognitive well-being.

Many studies underscore the cognitive advantages of physical activities. Regular physical exercise has been linked to improved executive function, better memory, and increased attention span (Hillman et al., 2008). These benefits are not only essential within the classroom setting but are transferrable skills that enhance everyday life. When children participate in sports or unstructured outdoor play, they learn decision-making, teamwork, and resilience. These experiences can significantly boost their cognitive and emotional resilience, preparing them for the challenges of our fast-paced digital world.

Blending digital play with physical activities can enhance learning experiences and make them more engaging and effective. For instance, augmented reality (AR) games that require children to move around their environment incorporate physical exercise seamlessly into digital play (Staiano & Calvert, 2011). These games often encourage players to explore their surroundings, transforming the entire world into a playground. Such technologies harness the appeal of digital play while simultaneously promoting physical activity.

The concept of gamification across various outdoor activities can redefine physical play for children who are particularly inclined towards digital experiences. Introducing elements of game design such as scores, badges, or levels to activities like hiking or cycling can motivate youngsters to participate and stay engaged. When blended correctly, this approach allows children to enjoy the merits of both digital and physical worlds without feeling forced to choose between the two.

Involving children in the selection of their physical activities can increase their motivation and commitment. Encouraging them to participate in team sports, individual activities like yoga or martial arts, or creative pursuits like dance or drama allows children to explore their passions and develop skills. Not every child will be inclined towards structured sports, hence providing diverse options ensures they find joy in physical activities that resonate with them personally.

Parents, educators, and caregivers should create environments that encourage a balance between screen time and outdoor play. Setting clear boundaries around digital use, such as designated technology-free times or areas, ensures that the focus remains on interactive physical play. These boundaries can help children learn the importance of moderation - a valuable lesson as they grow and gain independence.

The role of family and community in fostering this balance cannot be underestimated. Family hiking trips, community sports leagues, or organizing neighborhood friends for outdoor playdates demonstrates to children the value adults place on physical activity. It also serves to model healthy habits that they can carry into adulthood.

The interplay between digital technology and outdoor play also presents an opportunity for collaborative play and learning. Parents and caregivers might consider using digital tools that encourage outside exploration. Apps that identify plants or stars, or interactive games that require children to explore their neighborhoods, make outdoor play a shared adventure that incites curiosity and learning.

It is essential to recognize the social facets lost when children engage solely in digital play. Outdoor activities often require children to work together, building negotiation, conflict resolution, and communication skills. These social interactions, like agreeing on the rules of a game or learning to share equipment, contribute significantly to a child's emotional intelligence.

In conclusion, balancing outdoor play with digital interaction is possible and beneficial for children's holistic development. Parents and caregivers can achieve this equilibrium by creating supportive environments, setting boundaries, and providing varied and engaging opportunities for both types of play. As we move forward in this ever-evolving digital world, ensuring that the joys and benefits of the outdoors remain accessible and appealing to our children is crucial. It is in this balance that children can reap the full benefits of both worlds, nurturing their bodies, minds, and spirits for a healthier, more fulfilling life.

Setting Boundaries: How to Foster Healthy Gaming Habits in Kids & Teens

The vibrant world of video games offers a vast playground for kids and teens, full of opportunities for learning, fun, and social interaction. However, as with many aspects of digital life, moderation is key. While gaming can offer cognitive benefits like improved problem-solving skills and enhanced memory (Granic, Lobel, & Engels, 2014), excessive gaming has potential downsides, including social isolation and negative impacts on physical health. Setting boundaries is crucial in creating a balance that allows children to enjoy gaming's rewards without falling prey to its potential harms.

Start by setting clear rules around gaming time. The American Academy of Pediatrics suggests that children aged 6 and older should have no more than two hours of recreational screen time per day (AAP,

2016). Of course, these are just guidelines and need to be tailored to each child's needs and circumstances. For younger children, the time spent gaming should be even less, especially as they are still developing the skills to self-regulate. Schedule gaming sessions in a way that doesn't interfere with responsibilities like homework or chores, and especially not with sleep, which is essential for brain development and emotional regulation (Becker et al., 2016).

Involving kids in the process of setting these boundaries can be very effective. When children understand the reasons behind the limits, they are more likely to comply with them. Instead of framing it as restriction, emphasize balance. Discuss the importance of a variety of activities — from playing outside to reading books and engaging in family time. In this way, they learn to value moderation instead of feeling that their gaming privileges are arbitrarily taken away.

Another key aspect is the selection of games. Choose games that are age-appropriate and that offer educational or cognitive benefits. There are various parental guides and ratings, such as the ESRB ratings, that can help in selecting suitable games. Look for games that encourage creativity, problem-solving, or have social elements that can help develop teamwork and communication skills (Adachi & Willoughby, 2013).

Encouraging kids to play games offline is also a great way to foster healthy habits. Board games, puzzles, and outdoor sports can provide similar cognitive benefits without the potential drawbacks of screen time. Playing these games as a family not only limits digital exposure but also fosters communication and bonding, providing both emotional and cognitive benefits.

Empathy and communication are crucial in this process. Kids should feel comfortable discussing the games they enjoy and why they like them. Engage in conversations about their gaming experiences — what challenges did they face in a game, how did they overcome them?

This engagement shows them that you're interested in their world, which can lead to discussions about the challenges of excessive gaming, such as sleep problems or decreased academic performance.

Creating an environment where it feels safe to speak about the digital world invites open discussions about potential negative experiences, like online bullying or uncomfortable encounters. Children and teens should always feel able to approach adults for advice or help, knowing they won't be judged or punished for the discussion.

Technology has advanced rapidly and parenting in the digital age can seem daunting, but it offers many opportunities to guide new generations in swimming safely through the digital waters. By setting boundaries, choosing age-appropriate content, and staying engaged with kids' gaming experiences, you empower them to enjoy games in a healthy and balanced manner.

Ultimately, it's about nurturing their autonomy while keeping a safety net below to catch them when they might fall. With a blend of guidance and freedom, kids and teens can develop a relationship with gaming that's both enriching and balanced, contributing positively to their cognitive and emotional growth.

Chapter 11: The Impact of Digital Distraction on Brain Health & Safety

In today's fast-paced digital age, the omnipresence of screens and devices poses a unique challenge to children's cognitive and emotional development. With constant notifications, alerts, and the allure of social media, young minds are increasingly susceptible to digital distractions, which can fragment attention and impede learning. Research shows that the brain's neural pathways are highly adaptable during childhood, making this period crucial for fostering healthy focus and learning habits (Christakis, 2019). Yet, when faced with continuous digital interruptions, children may struggle to maintain deep concentration, a skill vital for academic and emotional success (Carr, 2010). Furthermore, the risks extend beyond the mental sphere, as distracted behaviors, such as the alarming uptick in "phone zombies" — pedestrians absorbed in their screens — can compromise physical safety (Nasr et al., 2021). By establishing clear and consistent screen boundaries at both home and school, parents and educators can cultivate environments that minimize digital distractions and support the balanced growth necessary for a thriving future. Encouraging practices like device-free zones and scheduled screen time not only protect young brains but also empower children to master the discipline of focus, paving the way to sustained cognitive and emotional well-being.

How Constant Notifications & Alerts Disrupt Focus & Learning

In today's fast-paced world, digital devices have become ubiquitous, and with them comes an avalanche of notifications and alerts that are a constant presence in our lives. This endless stream of pings and vibrations can have a profound impact on children's ability to focus and learn. Understanding the role of these digital interruptions is crucial as parents, teachers, and caregivers strive to support the cognitive and emotional development of the younger generation.

Imagine a classroom filled with eager students ready to learn, only to be disrupted intermittently by the chime of a notification. This scene is not imaginary; it's the reality for many children today. Research has shown that each time a notification is received, it can take substantial time for a person to regain their full concentration. The "switching cost" incurred when our attention shifts from a learning task to a notification is particularly detrimental to children whose executive functions are still developing (Bailey et al., 2018).

These interruptions are not just a matter of inconvenience but pose a real threat to learning efficiency. Each alert demands cognitive resources that would otherwise be devoted to absorbing information, solving problems, or thinking critically. This competition for attention can lessen the depth of learning and make it increasingly difficult for children to engage with academic content meaningfully. Moreover, frequent interruptions can stimulate a stress response, making it harder for the brain to associate learning with positive emotions. When learning becomes synonymous with stress, children might shy away from educational endeavors.

Scientific studies indicate that digital distractions have a direct impact on memory formation and recall. When the brain is interrupted by a notification, both working memory and the ability to transfer information into long-term storage are compromised. Without deep processing of information, memory retention falters, impacting the assimilation of knowledge necessary for both academic success and overall cognitive development (Karpinski et al., 2013).

From a neurological perspective, the developing brain of a child is particularly susceptible to the lure of notifications. The brain's reward centers light up at the sound of a new alert, releasing dopamine, the "feel-good" neurotransmitter that reinforces behaviors. This reinforcement can create a cycle where children feel compelled to attend to their devices, even when engaged in other tasks. Over time, this can contribute to increased impulsivity and decreased ability to focus, laying the groundwork for attention-related issues (Rosen et al., 2013).

Despite these challenges, it is possible to create an environment where digital distractions are minimized. Prioritizing notification-free periods, both in educational settings and at home, can help children maintain focus on the task at hand. Practical strategies include setting specific times for checking devices, creating physical spaces dedicated to digital-free activities, and using apps that limit screen time and block notifications during critical learning periods.

Teachers play a pivotal role in managing digital distractions in the classroom. By fostering a culture that values deep learning over multitasking, educators can help children develop the skills needed to manage their digital engagement. Teaching techniques such as mindfulness practices can encourage students to become more aware of their attention and the impact of interruptions. When students learn to recognize the prelude of a distraction, they can develop the metacognitive awareness necessary to manage their responses and maintain focus.

Likewise, parents and caregivers can reinforce these strategies at home. Establishing a balanced media diet and modeling mindful media use are critical. Children are observant of adult behaviors and are likely to replicate them. When caregivers prioritize face-to-face interactions and show restraint in their own media consumption, children learn to value presence and focus over constant digital engagement.

In light of these considerations, our challenge is to navigate a digital landscape without allowing it to overshadow the foundational aspects of learning and brain health. By understanding and mitigating the effects of constant notifications, we empower children to reclaim their attention and channel it towards growth, curiosity, and understanding. In doing so, we nurture a generation equipped not just with knowledge, but the ability to wield it in an ever-distracted world.

As we continue to explore the intersection of technology and education, it's clear that thoughtful intervention can transform potential disruptors into tools that support brain health rather than detract from it. By maintaining an awareness of our digital habits and fostering environments conducive to focused learning, we can ensure that children develop the resilience and cognitive abilities that are essential for lifelong success.

Walking While Distracted: The Rise of "Phone Zombies"

Walking while staring intently at a smartphone screen is now so pervasive that it's coined a term: "phone zombies". This phenomenon poses more than just a humorous image—it's a growing concern for public safety and personal well-being. From bustling city sidewalks to quieter suburban streets, the sight of individuals absorbed by their devices, often oblivious to their surroundings, is ever more common. But let's dig deeper into how this behavior impacts brain health and overall safety.

The issue of walking while distracted, especially by mobile devices, gains significance in the context of children and adolescents whose cognitive functions are still developing. Unlike adults, younger individuals are mastering skills such as spatial awareness and risk assessment. When kids walk with their eyes glued to a screen, they not only risk physical harm but also inhibit the natural development of these crucial skills (Strayer et al., 2013).

Why is this an alarming trend? For one, walking requires a continuous integration of sensory inputs and motor outputs—a process that smartphones interrupt. Research has shown that divided attention, such as that stemming from phone use while walking, can lead to slower obstacle avoidance and increased likelihood of stumbling or running into objects (Hyman et al., 2014). But the risks extend beyond mere physical injury; long-term cognitive impacts could also occur as children miss ongoing opportunities to engage their environments fully.

As parents, teachers, and caregivers, understanding these risks allows for the creation of interventions aimed at reducing the habitual nature of phone use while walking. We can encourage children to disconnect temporarily, focusing instead on their present physical environment. Such practices won't only ensure safety; they also enrich the growth of cognitive and spatial skills during a child's formative years.

One might wonder: what's so captivating on those small screens that it eclipses the immediate reality? The psychology behind this behavior is rooted in the allure of instant gratification and the human tendency to seek out information. Notifications, messages, and ever-updating social media feeds provide a dopamine hit that the real world finds difficult to replicate (Roberts et al., 2015). Ironically, the digital age, which means to connect us, is often a barrier to genuine human interaction.

We've observed firsthand how children, engrossed in their phones, tend to neglect or miss social cues and natural stimuli that are vital for the development of social intelligence and empathy. Think about a child walking home from school, sidelining potential interactions with peers or adults in the community in favor of digital engagement. Those moments provide real-world learning opportunities—learning that is disrupted when attention is diverted to a screen.

To tackle this rising issue, it's critical to promote awareness about the balance between digital consumption and real-world interaction. This isn't to demonize technology but to foster a healthier relationship with it. By allowing children and teenagers to set "tech-free" periods, especially during walks or commutes, we encourage them to engage with and appreciate their surroundings, thereby nurturing their cognitive and emotional growth.

Schools and community programs can also play a pivotal role in addressing this issue. Educational initiatives focusing on mindful gadget use can underscore the importance of being aware of one's physical environment. Simple practices like "tech down when you walk" can be taught as part of safety guidelines, much like looking both ways before crossing the street. This could extend to behavior modeling, wherein adults demonstrate responsible device use themselves.

There are innovative ways to integrate technology positively while circumventing the risks of turning into phone zombies. For instance, incorporate apps that promote physical and mental exercises in outdoor settings, or use augmented reality to encourage environmental interaction while being safely stationary. These methods bridge the gap between the digital and the tangible world, preserving the child's natural curiosity without compromising safety.

In short, while smartphones and other digital devices hold undeniable value in modern life, their use requires moderation, especially in contexts that demand full attention. By fostering environments that encourage active, real-world engagement, we can help children develop into well-rounded individuals who appreciate the world beyond the screen.

By understanding and addressing the dynamic between tech use and environmental awareness, we empower the next generation to harness technology wisely. And in doing so, we contribute positively to their cognitive and emotional well-being.

The Dangers of Texting & Driving for Teens (and Adults)

In today's fast-paced digital world, the urge to stay connected at all times can lead to dangerous habits, especially when behind the wheel. Texting and driving is not just a concern for teens; it's a perilous risk for adults, too. This form of digital distraction compromises brain health and safety, highlighting the urgent need to address its dangers and impact on individuals of all ages.

The statistics surrounding texting and driving are alarming. Studies show that teens are particularly susceptible, with motor vehicle accidents being the leading cause of death for this age group (Centers for Disease Control and Prevention, 2020). However, adults are not immune. The National Safety Council reported that in 2019, distracted driving caused over 3,000 fatalities in the United States alone (National Safety Council, 2020). Such numbers illustrate the stark reality that the simple act of sending a text message can have devastating consequences.

The neurological implications of texting while driving are profound. When individuals engage in this activity, their brains are thrust into a multitasking mode that's both inefficient and dangerous. Neuroscientific research suggests that the human brain cannot truly perform two high-level cognitive tasks simultaneously. Rather, it switches rapidly from one to the other, leading to lapses in attention and increased risk of errors (Just et al., 2008). When one of those tasks involves driving, the potential for catastrophic outcomes rises exponentially.

For teens, the consequences of texting and driving are compounded by developmental factors. Adolescent brains are still maturing, particularly in areas related to decision-making and impulse control (Giedd et al., 2015). As a result, teens may be more prone to engage in risky behaviors, underestimating the danger and overestimating their ability to handle distractions. This vulnerability necessitates targeted interventions and education aimed at both teens and their guardians.

Parents, teachers, and caregivers play a pivotal role in setting expectations and modeling safe behavior.

Effective strategies to combat texting and driving begin with open conversations focusing on its real dangers. Teens need to understand the science—how distractions hinder their reaction times and why this makes texting while driving so risky. Sharing real-life stories of accidents and tragedies caused by distracted driving can create a lasting impression and cement the seriousness of this behavior.

Moreover, practical measures can be implemented to reduce temptation. Encouraging the use of apps that block notifications while driving is one proactive step. Setting phones to "Do Not Disturb" or using driving-mode features can help ensure that incoming texts don't distract the driver. Parents should also establish clear household rules regarding phone use in cars, enforcing the idea that no message is worth risking lives over.

The role of education in schools cannot be overstated. Integrating programs that simulate the dangers of distracted driving provides experiential learning that words alone might fail to convey. By practicing response times in controlled environments, teens can experience firsthand how drastically distractions impact their ability to drive safely.

For adults, modeling appropriate behavior is crucial. Children and teens often learn by observing, so parents, teachers, and caregivers must exhibit the behavior they wish to see. By refraining from texting and driving and discussing their choices openly, adults reinforce the expectation that safety takes precedence over connectivity.

Public campaigns and community-based programs can further reinforce these lessons. Partnering with local law enforcement to hold talks and demonstrations or engaging in nationally recognized movements raises awareness on a broader scale. Communities need to cultivate a culture where the dangers of texting and driving are continuously re-emphasized, making it socially unacceptable.

While technology is part of the problem, it's also part of the solution. The development of hands-free technology and improvements in automotive safety features have the potential to mitigate risks. However, reliance on technology shouldn't overshadow the fundamental responsibility of drivers to remain focused and vigilant.

Addressing the dangers of texting and driving requires a multi-faceted approach. It involves education, legislation, and technology working hand in hand to foster safer habits on the road. For parents, teachers, and caregivers, the mission is clear: to support a generation that prioritizes lives over likes and understands the brain health and safety implications of their digital behaviors. Recognizing the urgency and acting upon it ensures that children are not only aware of the risks but are empowered to make smarter decisions.

How to Set Healthy Screen Boundaries at Home & School

In today's digital age, screens are everywhere. They're in our homes, schools, even in our pockets. While technology can be an invaluable educational tool, excessive screen time can disrupt a child's cognitive and emotional development. It's crucial for parents, teachers, and caregivers to establish healthy screen boundaries to ensure technology serves as a positive aid rather than a disruptive force.

Firstly, acknowledge the allure of screens. Digital devices are designed to capture and maintain attention with features like notifications, bright colors, and interactive elements. But this doesn't mean we must surrender to them. Setting boundaries starts with understanding the appeal of screens and communicating with children about their usage. Create a home and school environment where open conversations about screen time and its effects are normalized. Discuss with children how screens can affect concentration and encourage them to notice when their attention starts to wane.

Implementing clear, consistent rules about screen time is essential. At home, this might mean establishing tech-free zones, like the dining room or bedrooms, to encourage family interaction and healthier sleep habits. According to a study by Twenge et al. (2018), excessive screen time is linked to poor sleep quality, which can hinder cognitive function the next day. Set times for screen use, ensuring they align with family values and individual needs. For instance, permit screen time only after homework and chores are completed.

In schools, screen use should be directly tied to educational outcomes. Teachers set boundaries by integrating screens into lesson plans that enhance rather than replace traditional learning methods. It's important to blend digital tools with hands-on activities, encouraging students to connect their learning experiences with the real world. This balance helps students develop critical thinking skills and apply theoretical knowledge practically.

Moreover, it's not just about limiting time; it's also about monitoring content. Curate the kinds of apps, games, and shows that children are allowed to access. Educational content that promotes critical thinking and problem-solving is preferable. For example, software that supports STEM learning or language development can be beneficial. Encourage children to choose educational programs that spark their curiosity or creativity. This empowers them to make healthy screen choices on their own, reinforcing self-regulation skills.

Schedules should be flexible but firm. Life can be unpredictable, and sometimes screen time rules need to adapt. Occasional deviations are to be expected, but returning to established routines should be the goal. Positive reinforcement can be a powerful tool in maintaining these boundaries. Rewarding children for adhering to screen rules with extra playtime or a family activity can reinforce good habits.

Parental role modeling is vital. Children often emulate the behavior of adults, so it's important that parents and caregivers demonstrate controlled screen use. This means being mindful of one's own device time and showing children that screens are tools, not crutches. Encourage family activities that don't involve screens, like board games, hiking, or visiting a museum. Such activities not only break the screen cycle but also strengthen familial bonds and promote mental and emotional well-being.

Community involvement can bolster efforts at school. School administrators and teachers can work with parents to create consistent screen use guidelines across different settings. This could involve workshops or informational meetings where strategies for maintaining healthy digital environments are shared and refined. Leveraging the insights of educational and psychological experts can also provide compelling reasons to sustain these practices. When schools and families work together, the potential for positive changes in digital habits significantly increases.

Lastly, as we navigate the positives and pitfalls of technology, it's essential to remind ourselves and our children of the value of boredom. Allowing children moments without screens can stimulate creativity and problem-solving, fostering a sense of individual independence. As Siegel and Bryson (2011) point out, downtime empowers children to tap into their inner resources, developing deeper cognitive and emotional resilience.

In conclusion, setting healthy screen boundaries requires a thoughtful, strategic approach that combines clear rules, effective communication, and collaboration between home and school environments. By doing so, we're not only managing screen time effectively but actively supporting the cognitive and emotional development of children. In a world that constantly pulls towards the digital, ensuring balance is a step toward nurturing healthier, more well-rounded individuals.

Chapter 12: Digital Brain Training & Learning Programs for Kids

In our increasingly digital world, it's no surprise that kids' educational journeys have embraced technology, offering a host of digital brain training and learning programs aimed at enhancing cognitive skills. These digital tools, including apps and websites, promise to boost memory, focus, and learning capabilities through engaging interfaces and interactive experiences. While the effectiveness of such programs, like BrainHQ and Lumosity, is still debated among researchers, some studies suggest they can offer modest improvements in certain cognitive functions, particularly when used consistently and appropriately (Simons et al., 2016). However, it's crucial to approach these tools with a balanced mindset, considering the potential for overstimulation and the need for varied offline activities. As parents, teachers, and caregivers, embracing these digital aids means fostering not just technical proficiency but understanding the role of AI and gamification—elements that are shaping the future of education (Dede, 2010). By integrating these programs wisely into children's routines, we can cultivate a stimulating environment that complements traditional learning while aligning with their natural inclinations towards technology.

What Are Brain Training Games? Do They Work?

The concept of brain training games has gained remarkable popularity in recent years, especially among parents and educators eager to bolster the cognitive skills of children. These digital platforms, often marketed as enhancing memory, attention, and problem-solving skills, promise an engaging avenue of mental stimulation. But do they truly deliver on their claims? Understanding the potential and limitations of these games can help us make informed decisions about incorporating them into children's educational landscapes.

At their core, brain training games are designed to stimulate specific cognitive functions like memory, attention span, and problem-solving abilities. They are often structured as interactive puzzles or challenges that children can engage with on a computer, tablet, or smartphone. The appeal is clear: using games as a medium for learning can make cognitive exercises feel more like entertainment than schoolwork. This gamified experience is particularly beneficial in maintaining the engagement and motivation of young learners.

Several studies have delved into the efficacy of brain training games. Some suggest modest improvements in the skills directly targeted by these games. For instance, a child who plays memory enhancement games regularly might show some progress in short-term recall tasks (Simons et al., 2016). However, it's important to note that while specific functions may see improvement, the transfer of these skills to broader, real-world applications remains contentious. According to research by Owen et al. (2010), while brain training might improve performance on the trained tasks, there's little evidence these improvements extend to general cognitive capabilities or everyday tasks.

Moreover, the hype surrounding these games often overshadows a crucial aspect of cognitive development: the importance of a holistic approach. The brain doesn't operate in isolated compartments. Emotional development, physical health, and social interaction play equally pivotal roles in a child's cognitive growth. As such, relying solely on digital games for cognitive development overlooks these foundational elements. For example, engaging in physical activities can enhance a child's focus and executive functions (Hillman et al., 2014). Therefore, brain training games should be seen as a supplementary tool rather than a standalone solution.

However, it would be unjust to dismiss brain training games entirely. When thoughtfully incorporated into a child's routine, these games can complement traditional learning methods and other creative activities. For instance, pairing interactive games with reading or outdoor play can create a balanced cognitive engagement strategy. Encouragingly, several digital platforms are now aiming to integrate a wider variety of educational materials that consider emotional and social learning alongside cognitive skills.

Another essential aspect to consider is the customization potential offered by digital brain training tools. Unlike traditional learning, where curriculums can be rigid, digital games can adapt their difficulty level and content based on the child's performance. This adaptability promotes a personalized learning experience that can cater to individual learning curves, ensuring that children remain challenged but not overwhelmed. Carefully selecting games that allow for such customization can maximize their benefits.

Moreover, these games can offer a window into a child's unique cognitive strengths and areas for improvement. By observing which games a child naturally excels in or struggles with, parents and educators can gather insights into a child's learning profile. This information can be invaluable when designing broader educational and support strategies, ensuring that other aspects of the child's education complement their cognitive development effectively.

On a cautionary note, the digital nature of brain training games also introduces potential downsides. Excessive screen time is a concern, particularly when it comes to the developing brains of children. The American Academy of Pediatrics recommends a balanced approach, emphasizing the need for direct human interaction and physical play alongside digital engagement. Over-reliance on screens, even for educational purposes, can lead to issues like reduced face-to-face social interactions and a more sedentary lifestyle, both of which are detrimental to holistic development.

In conclusion, brain training games can serve as one of many tools to support cognitive development. However, they shouldn't overshadow the significance of physical activity, social connections, and emotional well-being in a child's overall growth. These digital tools should be integrated thoughtfully and used as part of a diversified strategy that includes various learning experiences. Finally, ongoing research and responsible media use practices will be crucial in optimizing the role of brain training games in education, helping them evolve alongside our understanding of the intricate workings of the child's brain.

Comparing Popular Digital Learning Tools (BrainHQ, Lumosity, etc.)

In today's digital world, numerous apps and programs promise to enhance cognitive abilities and foster learning through games and exercises specifically designed for brain development. Parents, educators, and caregivers are inundated with options, but selecting the right tool requires understanding their benefits and limitations. This section dives into the comparative analysis of popular digital learning tools such as BrainHQ and Lumosity, focusing on their effectiveness, unique features, and appropriateness for children's evolving cognitive needs.

BrainHQ and Lumosity stand out as two of the most recognized brain training tools, each offering a suite of exercises developed by neuroscientists. These tools aim to challenge the brain through tasks that claim to improve memory, attention, and problem-solving skills ("BrainHQ," 2023). But do they truly deliver on their promises? A critical look at the scientific backing behind these tools suggests that while they may offer some cognitive benefits, the results can vary widely among individuals. Research published in the Proceedings of the National Academy of Sciences indicates that while brain training can enhance certain aspects of cognitive function, its effects are not universally transformative and may not significantly transfer to real-world skills (Redick et al., 2013).

BrainHQ, developed by Posit Science, emphasizes personalized brain training exercises that adapt as the user progresses. This adaptability means that exercises can adjust difficulty levels based on a child's performance, potentially keeping them engaged and challenged. The program focuses on core cognitive skills, offering exercises that promote brain plasticity, which is crucial during childhood developmental stages. Similarly, Lumosity has a user-friendly interface gamifying cognitive exercises that target various mental domains ("Lumosity," 2023). While these tools offer a playful approach that can keep children entertained, parental guidance remains essential to ensure that screen time aligns with healthy habits.

Parents often wonder whether the investment in these tools translates to tangible educational benefits. Studies suggest that brain training can lead to modest improvements in specific cognitive skills, but these improvements might not necessarily translate to academic performance or other life skills (Simons et al., 2016). This revelation brings to light an important aspect of selecting digital learning tools: they should not be solely relied on for cognitive development. Instead, they can be an adjunct to a well-rounded regimen that includes physical activity, balanced nutrition, and sufficient sleep.

While both BrainHQ and Lumosity provide structured cognitive exercises, they differ in how these are delivered. Lumosity, for instance, places a significant emphasis on entertainment and fun, with visually appealing games that often feel like puzzles. BrainHQ, on the other hand, might appeal more to users looking for a serious commitment to improve cognitive functions, with exercises that feel more clinical but potentially more targeted (Hardy et al., 2015). This distinction is crucial for caregivers and educators when deciding which tool fits better into a child's learning ecosystem.

Moreover, the role of these tools in enhancing emotional and social skills is often debated. While primarily focused on cognitive development, they tend to overlook the broader spectrum of skills like emotional intelligence and social interaction capabilities. These are best developed through real-world interactions, play, and discussion, areas where even the most interactive digital programs fall short. For holistic development, digital tools should complement human interaction and experiential learning, not replace them.

Besides BrainHQ and Lumosity, many other tools are emerging with their unique claims and methodologies. However, the overarching consensus is that scientific validation and parental involvement are paramount. The involvement of an adult can guide the type of content and the duration of engagement, ensuring that these tools are being used effectively and safely. Considering the potential overreliance on technology, it is critical to strike a balance that doesn't lead to passive consumption but active engagement and learning.

In summary, while brain training tools like BrainHQ and Lumosity offer innovative ways to engage children cognitively, they must be used judiciously within a larger context of cognitive development strategies. The true power of these tools lies not in their ability to replace traditional learning and interaction but in enhancing and supplementing them. Digital learning tools can be valuable allies in supporting cognitive growth, providing they are part of a balanced and mindful developmental approach.

AI & Gamification in Education: The Future of Brain-Boosting Tech

As technology continues to evolve, AI and gamification are becoming integral components of educational programs designed to boost cognitive development in children. With their potential to personalize learning experiences and encourage active engagement, these tools hold promise in supporting both cognitive and emotional development. But what do these terms really mean, and how can they be harnessed effectively in educational settings?

Artificial intelligence (AI) refers to computer systems capable of performing tasks that typically require human intelligence, such as recognizing patterns or solving problems. In an educational context, AI can personalize learning by assessing a child's unique learning style and progress, subsequently adapting the content to meet individual needs. Imagine a system that can levy real-time assessments and adjust the difficulty of tasks according to a student's understanding. Such systems could potentially level the playing field, offering tailored support to every child, whether they're gifted or have specific learning challenges (Luckin et al., 2016).

Gamification, on the other hand, involves integrating game elements into non-game settings, like education. This technique is used to make learning more engaging and fun, often enhancing motivation and participation through the use of points, badges, or leaderboards. While some might worry about the superficial nature of rewards, gamification's true power lies in its ability to make the educational process enjoyable and immersive, sparking genuine interest and sustained attention (Dicheva et al., 2015).

The combination of AI and gamification can create a dynamic learning environment that adapts to the child's developmental needs, promoting active engagement while providing a rewarding experience. For instance, AI can identify a child's strengths and areas for improvement, guiding them through gamified learning paths that entice and challenge them appropriately. This approach can be particularly beneficial for children with attention difficulties or specific learning disabilities, offering tailored strategies that traditional methods might overlook.

Scientific research suggests that well-designed educational games can improve memory, attention, and other executive functions in children. For example, games that require players to memorize patterns or strategize their next moves can enhance working memory and problem-solving skills. These cognitive gains can extend beyond the game itself, supporting academic achievements and everyday decision-making (Granic et al., 2014). However, it's important for educators and parents to scrutinize the quality and intent of digital content, choosing tools that genuinely promote learning over those simply offering rewards.

One of the most exciting prospects of AI in education is its ability to provide instant feedback and personalized support. This real-time insight can lead to improved learning outcomes, as children receive the necessary guidance to overcome challenges and reinforce their understanding. Imagine a child struggling with math concepts; an AI-powered educational app could offer step-by-step problem-solving techniques, tailored hints, and alternative methods of explanation until the child reaches mastery. Such immediate and personalized intervention can preserve the child's confidence and curiosity, fostering a lifelong love for learning.

Moreover, AI's capability to track and analyze vast amounts of data opens up new avenues for understanding educational success. Educators can leverage these insights to refine teaching methods, curricula, and even classroom layouts. With a data-driven understanding of how and why children learn, educators can craft educational experiences that cater to diverse needs, supporting all facets of a child's development.

While the potential benefits are significant, adopting AI and gamification in education also demands caution. Over-reliance on technology could lead to diminished critical thinking and creativity, as children might become more accustomed to AI-driven solutions rather than engaging in original thought. It is crucial to strike a balance, ensuring that technology complements rather than replaces traditional learning methods. Incorporating AI and gamification should encourage inquiry and exploration, complementing face-to-face interactions and hands-on experiences that are vital for holistic development.

Another concern is equitable access to technology. AI and gamification, although promising, require resources and infrastructure that may not be available to all students, particularly those in underfunded schools or regions without robust internet connectivity. Addressing these disparities should be a priority, as equal access to learning tools is fundamental to ensuring that every child can benefit from technological advancements in education.

Ultimately, the goal is to create an educational environment where technology serves as a tool for exploration, creativity, and personalized learning. By combining the intuitive nature of AI with the engaging aspects of gamification, educational programs can offer rich, adaptable experiences that cater to individual learning needs. When implemented thoughtfully and responsibly, AI and gamification not only stimulate cognitive growth but also nurture the emotional and social skills essential for thriving in an increasingly complex world.

As parents, teachers, and caregivers strive to support children's cognitive and emotional development, it is important to stay informed and critically engaged with new educational technologies. By understanding and evaluating the role of AI and gamification, adults can better navigate the myriad of learning tools available, choosing those that best foster growth, curiosity, and well-being.

Educational stakeholders need to collaborate, share insights, and develop guidelines ensuring that AI and gamification are used ethically and effectively. This collaborative effort can include policymakers crafting regulations for safe and equal access, tech developers focusing on learner-friendly designs, and educators employing best practices for integration in classrooms. Working together, society can better leverage these technologies, paving the way for an enriched educational landscape that prioritizes the holistic development of every child.

In summary, AI and gamification in education present exciting opportunities for enhancing learning experiences, tailored to the varied needs of children. By prioritizing balanced integration, equitable access, and thoughtful evaluation, we can harness the potential of these technologies to cultivate well-rounded individuals ready to face the challenges of tomorrow. The future of brain-boosting tech is promising, pointing to a world where every child's educational journey is as engaging and effective as possible.

Apps, Websites, & Interactive Tools for Memory, Focus, & Learning

In today's digital cra, the landscape of learning tools has transformed substantially, offering a plethora of apps, websites, and interactive platforms designed to enhance children's cognitive skills. When used judiciously, these digital resources can serve as an effective supplement to traditional learning methods, offering pathways to enhance memory, focus, and overall learning capacity. The kcy is navigating these digital waters mindfully, ensuring that children engage with content that nurtures their cognitive and emotional development.

One significant advantage of digital learning tools is their adaptability to individual learning styles and paces. Interactive apps like

Khan Academy Kids offer personalized learning experiences, allowing children to explore subjects at their own pace, while receiving immediate feedback. This kind of tailored learning opportunity isn't just beneficial; it is vital in cultivating a child's intrinsic motivation and curiosity about the world around them (Lauricella et al., 2015). Through gamified elements, these platforms make learning engaging, turning the acquisition of knowledge into a delightful experience for young minds.

Memory and focus are two cognitive areas where digital tools can provide substantial support. Apps such as CogniFit and Peak are specifically designed to boost memory through a variety of brain-training games. These apps use adaptive algorithms to scale difficulty according to the child's progress, thereby continuously challenging their memory and concentration capabilities (Butler & Paul, 2019). Such adaptive features ensure that the brain is actively engaged, leading to improvements in neural efficiency and cognitive resilience over time.

Web-based tools also play a crucial role in modern learning environments. Websites like National Geographic Kids and NASA's Space Place offer captivating and educational content that can enrich what children learn in school. These platforms provide a wealth of videos, articles, and interactive games that make complex subjects more accessible and fascinating, aiding in both comprehension and retention. Furthermore, these resources encourage exploratory learning—a critical component of critical thinking and problem-solving development (Lemke et al., 2011).

Interactive tools that focus on developing emotional intelligence also deserve attention. Tools like Positive Penguins and Smiling Mind offer mindfulness exercises and emotional regulation strategies for children. These platforms help kids identify their emotions and learn coping strategies, which are crucial skills for emotional well-being and focus in academic settings. Such tools underscore the importance of balancing cognitive training with emotional health, ensuring that children grow into well-rounded individuals capable of managing life's challenges effectively.

The advent of AI and machine learning has only refined the capabilities of educational apps and websites, introducing more sophisticated tracking and adaptation of the learning process. Systems like DreamBox Learning employ AI to analyze the responsiveness of children to various content forms, enabling the platform to adapt lessons in real-time. The result is a highly personalized learning journey that keeps kids both challenged and motivated, tapping into the potential of every learner (Shute & Ke, 2012).

However, the use of digital tools must be balanced with offline activities. While leveraging apps and websites for educational purposes, it's essential to maintain a healthy balance with physical activities, social interactions, and non-digital play. The synergy between digital tools and real-world experiences is what ultimately optimizes children's cognitive and emotional growth. Parents and educators should set clear boundaries on screen time and guide children towards content that supports not just cognitive gains but also creativity and social skills.

Schools and educators can further support this balance by incorporating interactive tools into the classroom setting under guided supervision. This not only ensures that the tools are being used effectively but also that children are collaborating and engaging in social learning scenarios. Teachers can utilize platforms like Google Classroom and Edmodo to reinforce digital and social literacy concurrently, preparing students for a world that increasingly straddles the physical and digital realms.

While the integration of technology in education poses potential challenges—a key one being screen time—the benefits of judiciously used digital learning tools significantly outweigh the drawbacks. By augmenting traditional learning settings with well-selected digital tools, we pave the way for enriched learning experiences that cater to diverse needs and preferences, laying a strong foundation for lifelong learning in children.

Chapter 13: Recognizing When Professional Help is Needed

In the journey of nurturing a child's cognitive and emotional development, discerning when professional intervention is necessary is pivotal. Children possess unique developmental trajectories and, while parents, teachers, and caregivers can provide robust support through nutrition, sleep, movement, and mental exercises, at times, the signs of learning disabilities, developmental delays, or emotional struggles require more specialized attention. It's crucial to observe indicators such as consistent academic difficulties, marked behavioral changes, or emotional expressions that seem beyond the norm for their age. Promptly consulting with neurologists, pediatric psychologists, or other specialists can offer invaluable insights and tailored interventions to foster healthier outcomes (American Academy of Pediatrics, 2021). Emphasizing a proactive approach recognizes the importance of integrating professional expertise while continuing the everyday nurturing activities that bolster children's growth across all dimensions—cognitive, emotional, and social (Elias et al., 1997). Understanding professional help as an extension of caregiving strengthens the ecosystem supporting children, empowering adults to remain steadfast advocates for their well-being.

Signs of Learning Disabilities, Developmental Delays, or Emotional Struggles

Understanding the signs of learning disabilities, developmental delays, or emotional struggles is crucial for those who care for and support children. These challenges can manifest in various ways, and recognizing them early can significantly impact a child's future development and well-being. While each child is unique, some common indicators may suggest that professional help is warranted.

Learning disabilities often become apparent when a child struggles with reading, writing, or math, despite receiving adequate instruction and encouragement. These difficulties are not necessarily indicative of a lack of effort or intelligence but rather a distinct way in which the child's brain processes information. For instance, dyslexia, a common learning disability, affects reading abilities, making it hard for children to decode words and comprehend text (Lyon et al., 2003). Teachers and parents might notice persistent spelling mistakes, trouble remembering sequences, or difficulty understanding rhymes and phonics. Such observations may indicate the need for further evaluation by a specialist in educational psychology.

In terms of developmental delays, the signs are often detectable at a young age. Missing key milestones like walking, talking, or even nonverbal communication indicators, such as facial expressions and gestures, might suggest deeper underlying issues. Sensorimotor integration problems—difficulty in using the senses and motor skills together—can affect a child's ability to engage with their environment fully. Such developmental challenges often require the attention of a pediatrician or developmental specialist who can conduct a comprehensive assessment and outline suitable intervention strategies (Boyd et al., 2013).

Emotional struggles in children can be more challenging to pinpoint. However, certain behaviors can serve as red flags. Persistent sadness, withdrawal from social interactions, heightened anxiety, or intense, inappropriate emotional reactions may suggest emotional health issues. Sometimes these are situational, arising from changes in the child's environment, such as family disputes or school transitions. Other times, they may indicate conditions like anxiety disorders or depression, requiring the expertise of a child psychologist or psychiatrist (Emerson & Hatton, 2007).

It's important to approach these issues with empathy and patience. Each child's emotional and cognitive landscape is unique, and their struggles, whether apparent or subtle, can have profound impacts on their self-esteem and social interactions. Maintaining open lines of communication between children, parents, and educators is key to understanding the full scope of these challenges and their effects.

Collaboration among caregivers and professionals can lead to tailored interventions that suit the specific needs of the child. These interventions often include a combination of therapeutic approaches such as individualized education plans (IEPs), occupational therapy, speech therapy, and behavior modification techniques. For emotional struggles, cognitive-behavioral therapy (CBT) has been proven effective in helping children alter negative thought patterns and improve emotional regulation (Beck, 2011).

Early intervention is vital. Studies have shown that children who receive support for learning disabilities or developmental delays at an early stage are more likely to achieve better long-term outcomes, academically and socially (Landa, 2008). Being proactive not only alleviates current struggles but also sets the stage for a more confident and independent future.

That said, the journey to seeking professional help should be free of stigma. Encouraging a positive narrative around mental health and learning challenges both at home and in educational settings fosters an atmosphere where seeking help becomes a normalized part of a child's development. This cultural shift is significant in ensuring children have the courage to express their struggles and request the help they need.

For caregivers, understanding these signs and taking prompt action reflects a commitment to nurturing every facet of a child's growth. With the right support and intervention, children can develop into resilient and capable individuals, ready to face the complexities of the world with confidence.

In conclusion, caregivers must stay vigilant and informed. Recognizing the signs of learning disabilities, developmental delays, or emotional struggles is the first step. Seeking timely and appropriate professional help not only aids in the child's immediate development but also lays a foundation for future success and well-being.

When to Seek Cognitive or Behavioral Therapy

Recognizing the moment when a child's struggles go beyond the typical ups and downs of development can feel daunting for parents, teachers, and caregivers. It's essential to first acknowledge that seeking cognitive or behavioral therapy isn't an admission of failure; rather, it's a proactive step toward fostering a child's optimal growth. Therapy can offer tailored solutions that address unique challenges, empowering children to thrive emotionally and cognitively.

Children can face a myriad of challenges that affect their cognitive and emotional development. From difficulty keeping up with academic demands to struggling with peer interactions, the signs that a child might benefit from professional help can vary significantly. Often, the key indicator lies in persistence and severity. For instance, if a child experiences ongoing issues that disrupt everyday activities, or when difficulties seem to worsen over time, it might be time to explore professional intervention.

The process of identifying cognitive or behavioral therapy as a suitable option should involve careful observation and documentation of the child's behavior patterns. This includes monitoring how they respond to different stimuli and their interactions with others. Parents and educators should look for signs such as abrupt mood changes, prolonged sadness, excessive worry, difficulty concentrating, or noticeable declines in school performance. While occasional mood swings or temporary periods of stress are normal, persistent symptoms may warrant further evaluation.

Consulting with a pediatrician can serve as a valuable first step. Health professionals can conduct preliminary screenings and, if necessary, refer families to specialists in child psychology or psychiatry. It's crucial to involve a team approach where caregivers and professionals work closely together, ensuring the child receives comprehensive care. Open communication between parents, teachers, and therapists is essential to tailor the intervention effectively.

An essential consideration when seeking therapy is understanding the different modalities available. Cognitive-behavioral therapy (CBT) is one of the most common approaches. It's evidence-based and focuses on identifying and altering negative thought patterns and behaviors. CBT can help children develop coping strategies, improve emotional regulation, and enhance their problem-solving skills (Friedberg, McClure, & Garcia, 2009).

Apart from CBT, play therapy can be especially beneficial for younger children. This method leverages play as a natural medium for children to express themselves and work through their issues. Through guided play sessions, children can explore their thoughts and emotions in a safe and supportive environment. Play therapy can be an excellent way to reveal hidden emotions and thoughts that children might not discuss openly (Landreth, 2012).

In some instances, family therapy may also be recommended, particularly when the child's issues are closely linked with family dynamics. This approach helps to address concerns within the family system, fostering healthier communication patterns and stronger emotional bonds. By involving the entire family, children receive the support they need not just from a therapist, but from their home environment as well.

It is essential to trust instincts when considering therapy. Parents and caregivers often possess an intuitive understanding of their child's needs and can sense when something isn't quite right. Even when faced with doubts or societal stigma regarding therapy, it's important to prioritize the child's well-being. Seeking help is a step towards providing children with the tools they need to better understand themselves and navigate their world.

While the decision to seek therapy can be unsettling, it is often accompanied by great rewards. Therapy empowers children by offering them a safe space to articulate their experiences and emotions. It provides them with strategies to manage stress, bolster self-esteem, and develop resilience. These skills are invaluable, supporting not just immediate needs but fostering lifelong emotional health and cognitive function.

Parents, educators, and caregivers should remain vigilant, open-minded, and prepared to act when necessary. Recognizing when to seek professional help is not just about addressing present challenges; it's about investing in a child's future, ensuring they have the foundation to lead a balanced and fulfilling life. After all, the ultimate goal is to nurture children who can think critically, interact positively, and feel secure in their environment.

Understanding the Role of Neurologists, Pediatric Psychologists, and Other Specialists

Sometimes, understanding and supporting a child's cognitive and emotional development requires more than just parental intuition and dedication. While parents, teachers, and caregivers are invaluable in nurturing a child's growth, there are instances where specialized expertise becomes essential. This is where professionals like neurologists and pediatric psychologists come into play, providing insights and interventions that can significantly impact a child's development for the better.

Neurologists, for example, are doctors trained in the diagnosis and treatment of nervous system disorders, which include the brain. When it comes to children's development, they play a crucial role, especially if there are observable signs of neurological issues. If a child shows symptoms such as persistent headaches, unexplained seizures, or developmental delays, a neurologist can conduct various tests to pinpoint or rule out conditions like epilepsy or developmental disorders. Having a professional identify and treat potential neurological problems promptly can make a difference in managing or even completely resolving such issues. Their expertise not only provides a clear understanding of the condition but also helps in creating a tailored plan that optimizes the child's development and quality of life (Rosenbaum & Leviton, 1996).

Moreover, pediatric psychologists are invaluable when it comes to addressing a child's emotional and behavioral development. These professionals focus on understanding and improving the psychological well-being of children and adolescents. They work with children who may experience anxiety, depression, or behavioral problems and employ evidence-based therapies to guide them towards emotional balance and coping strategies. If a child is struggling emotionally or behaviorally, seeing a pediatric psychologist can help identify underlying issues that may not be apparent to the parent or teacher. Interventions might include cognitive-behavioral therapy or family counseling, which aim to equip children and their families with the tools needed to improve mental health and interpersonal dynamics (Mash & Wolfe, 2019).

In some cases, occupational therapists and speech-language pathologists may also be part of a child's support team. These specialists address specific areas of a child's development. Occupational therapists help children who battle with fine motor skills, feeding issues, or sensory processing disorders. By utilizing targeted exercises and activities, they can help strengthen a child's ability to perform daily tasks and engage socially. Meanwhile, speech-language pathologists focus on addressing speech or language delays, working with kids to improve their communication skills. Whether it's a stutter or difficulties in understanding language, their intervention can be pivotal in overcoming these hurdles, thus supporting both academic achievement and social interaction (American Speech-Language-Hearing Association, 2021).

Collaboration among these experts often leads to the most effective outcomes. For instance, if a child is diagnosed with ADHD, a neurologist might oversee medical treatments while a pediatric psychologist works on behavioral strategies. An occupational therapist might contribute exercises to improve focus and sensory integration. This multidisciplinary approach ensures that the child receives comprehensive care addressing different facets of their development. Such a synergy highlights how intertwined these specialties are when it comes to understanding complexities in child development.

It's also important for parents and teachers to understand the role of these specialists to avoid unnecessary anxiety. The thought of involving specialists can sometimes be intimidating due to misconceptions or fear of stigma. However, seeking professional help should be viewed as a proactive step towards empowerment, providing children with the right environment to thrive and develop optimally. Specialists offer insights and interventions that are often transformative, ensuring that any underlying issues do not interfere with the child's growth (Thomas & Chess, 1977).

Ultimately, recognizing when it's time to consult a specialist is a critical component of supporting a child's cognitive and emotional development. While the signs may vary from child to child, being attuned to persistent issues that seem beyond the scope of routine parenting or teaching is crucial. With professionals' help, children not only get the support they need to overcome hurdles but also the opportunity to unlock their full potential in both cognitive and emotional domains.

As parents, teachers, and caregivers, it is invaluable to maintain open communication with these specialists and be part of the conversation about the child's progress and challenges. Understanding each role these professionals play helps in forging effective partnerships, ensuring that all interventions align with the child's unique needs and circumstances. Recognizing the importance of each specialist allows us to better prepare ourselves in guiding children through their diverse developmental journeys, leaving room for expertise when it counts.

Appendix A: Appendix & Further Resources

This appendix serves as a comprehensive guide for parents, teachers, and caregivers who aim to nurture children's cognitive and emotional development through brain-friendly habits. Included are thoughtfully curated books for various age groups, encompassing engaging fiction and enlightening nonfiction that promote brain growth. Dive into additional reading material and scientific studies that provide deeper insights into childhood brain development (Giedd et al., 2009). Explore recommended apps and learning games designed to stimulate the mind while being mindful of healthy screen time practices. Gain access to nutritional guidelines, featuring sample meal plans focused on brain-boosting nutrition, ensuring that children are fueled for optimal thinking and emotional balance (Fernandes et al., 2020). Furthermore, find essential contacts and guidelines for recognizing when professional assistance is needed, alongside easy ways to connect with support organizations for learning disabilities, ADHD, and emotional health. Each resource aims to empower you in creating a balanced environment that fosters resilience and intellectual growth, steering clear of negative influences (Sunderland, 2007).

Recommended Books for Different Age Groups (Brain-Boosting Fiction & Nonfiction)

It's no secret that reading is one of the most powerful tools for cognitive and emotional development. Not only does reading provide a gateway to new worlds and ideas, but it also enhances various brain functions and emotional skills (Neuman & Celano, 2012). What follows is a carefully curated list of fiction and nonfiction books tailored to different age groups, with the intent to foster a lifelong love of reading and learning.

For Infants and Toddlers (Ages 0-3):

At this tender age, books with vibrant pictures and simple text are crucial. They help infants understand language and recognize familiar objects. One standout is "Goodnight Moon" by Margaret Wise Brown. This classic bedtime story's soothing rhythm helps forge emotional connections while supporting language development. Another gem is "The Very Hungry Caterpillar" by Eric Carle, which combines counting, days of the week, and a tale of transformation, offering a holistic developmental boost (Carle, 1969).

Interactive books, like "Pat the Bunny" by Dorothy Kunhardt, with its texture elements, are also beneficial. They not only keep little fingers engaged but also develop sensory skills. For nonfiction, try "Whose Baby am I?" by John Butler. It's a great way to introduce young toddlers to the animal kingdom.

For Preschoolers (Ages 3-5):

Books at this stage start to introduce more complex language and themes. "Where the Wild Things Are" by Maurice Sendak is not just a journey into the imagination but also explores emotions such as anger and reconciliation. It helps preschoolers understand their feelings in a safe environment (Sendak, 1963).

Nonfiction options, like "National Geographic Little Kids First Big Book of Why" by Amy Shields, open the door to curiosity about the world. It's full of incredible facts about nature, science, and everyday phenomena that encourage inquisitiveness.

For Early Elementary (Ages 5-8):

This age group can delight in stories where they start seeing themselves reflected in different characters and scenarios. "Charlotte's Web" by E.B. White is a classic tale of friendship and sacrifice, perfect for this age. It not only enriches vocabulary but also imbues valuable life lessons (White, 1952).

For nonfiction enthusiasts, "The Magic School Bus" series by Joanna Cole and Bruce Degen can satisfy the curiosity of young minds about various scientific topics. Each book is like a mini-exploration into fields like the human body, outer space, and the ecosystem.

For Tweens (Ages 9-12):

As children grow, their appetite for complex narratives and knowledge deepens. "Harry Potter and the Sorcerer's Stone" by J.K. Rowling provides an imaginative journey and explores concepts of courage, friendship, and perseverance. The series not only strengthens syntax comprehension but also introduces mythological and literary references (Rowling, 1997).

For nonfiction that challenges them, "Bomb: The Race to Build—and Steal—the World's Most Dangerous Weapon" by Steve Sheinkin offers a gripping scientific history. It teaches about real-world events with accuracy and engagement, perfect for developing critical thinking skills.

For Teens (Ages 13-18):

This stage benefits from literature that critically engages with identity and society. "To Kill a Mockingbird" by Harper Lee is essential reading for discussing issues of race, justice, and moral growth. It promotes empathy and societal awareness, essential components of emotional intelligence (Lee, 1960).

For the non-fictional mind, "The 7 Habits of Highly Effective Teens" by Sean Covey offers practical wisdom. It's an adaptation from the popular adult version that's accessible enough for teenagers to form healthy habits propelling their personal growth and future success.

Ultimately, each of these books serves a purpose—whether it's to entertain, educate, or elicit deep thinking. By tailoring book selections to the developmental needs and interests of each age group, we not only promote brain development but also instill a love for lifelong learning and cognitive resilience.

Additional Reading & Scientific Studies (Books, Research Papers, Trusted Websites)

For those interested in delving deeper into the captivating world of children's cognitive and emotional development, a wealth of literature offers both empirical research and practical guidance. Books by renowned psychologists and neurologists provide insights into how children's brains grow and adapt. Resources like research papers and trusted websites can be incredibly useful in expanding your knowledge base.

A fantastic starting point is "The Whole-Brain Child" by Daniel J. Siegel and Tina Payne Bryson. This book bridges the gap between scientific understanding and practical application, illustrating how parents can nurture optimal brain development. Siegel and Bryson emphasize strategies that integrate the brain's different regions, facilitating balanced and healthy development. Their work is well-grounded in contemporary neuroscience and offers a user-friendly approach to incorporating these insights into everyday parenting practices.

For a deeper dive into how children's minds develop from a psychological perspective, Carol Dweck's "Mindset: The New Psychology of Success" remains essential reading. Dweck distinguishes between fixed and growth mindsets, explaining how our beliefs about abilities can profoundly influence how children learn and handle challenges. Her research underlies many educational strategies aimed at fostering resilience and a love of learning, making it an invaluable resource for parents and educators alike.

Research papers provide another layer of understanding, offering detailed studies on various aspects of developmental psychology, neuroplasticity, and educational psychology. One noteworthy paper is "The Role of Sleep in Emotional Brain Function" by Walker and van der Helm (2009), which examines how sleep affects emotional regulation and memory consolidation in children and adolescents. Understanding these processes helps caregivers create effective sleep routines that support cognitive and emotional health, aligning with the practices outlined in this book's section on sleep.

Another intriguing area of study is the impact of movement and exercise on brain development. Coe et al. (2006) present groundbreaking findings in "The Relationship Between Physical Activity, Cognitive Function, and Academic Achievement in Children," highlighting how exercise can enhance concentration, memory, and even classroom behavior. This study underscores the connection between physical activity and cognitive performance, providing solid evidence for encouraging active play as part of a balanced approach to child development.

For digital resources, the website of the Center on the Developing Child at Harvard University offers comprehensive data and insights on early childhood brain development. Their resources are meticulously curated, providing accessible but scientifically rigorous information for parents, caregivers, and educators. Topics range from the foundational principles of brain architecture to how stress can impact developing minds.

The American Academy of Pediatrics (AAP) is another vital online resource. The AAP's guidelines and research papers give evidence-based advice on topics such as screen time, nutrition, and sleep, reflecting the latest scientific consensus. They offer practical tips to ensure children engage with digital media healthily and productively, dovetailing with the strategies addressed in the chapters on screen time and digital play.

It's equally important to seek data from longitudinal studies, which track development over time and provide unique insights into how early interventions can yield long-lasting benefits. The renowned Dunedin Study, for example, has followed participants since birth and delivered key findings on a range of developmental outcomes, from health to cognitive performance. Such studies reveal the long-term effectiveness of early life influences on brain development, supporting the approaches advocated throughout this book.

When it comes to neuroplasticity—the brain's incredible ability to reorganize itself in response to learning and experience—works by Michael Merzenich are pivotal. Known as one of the pioneers in the field, Merzenich's research elucidates how targeted mental exercises can enhance cognitive function, debunking the myth that brain development halts after a certain age. His findings are laid out in "Soft-Wired: How the New Science of Brain Plasticity Can Change Your Life," which is particularly valuable for those interested in harnessing brain plasticity strategies geared towards both children and adults.

Finally, trusted websites like the National Institute of Child Health and Human Development (NICHD) offer a plethora of reliable and valid information. The NICHD covers topics including childhood nutrition and its impact on growth and cognitive development, essentials that align with the robust nutritional guidelines emphasized in our discussion on brain-boosting foods.

Engaging with these readings and resources will not only enhance your understanding but equip you with practical strategies for fostering an environment conducive to healthy brain development. By staying informed through a blend of books, research papers, and digital content, you'll be well-prepared to support and nurture the developmental needs of the children in your care.

Recommended Brain-Boosting Apps & Learning Games for Kids

In today's digital age, technology, when used thoughtfully, can be a powerful ally in enhancing children's cognitive and emotional development. With a plethora of apps and learning games available, it's possible to provide intellectually engaging and developmentally appropriate content that complements traditional learning methods. Before diving into specific recommendations, it's important to understand that not all digital experiences are created equal. Parents, teachers, and caregivers should seek out digital tools that prioritize educational content, foster creativity, and avoid overstimulation.

One highly acclaimed app is *Endless Alphabet*, which is ideal for young learners. Designed for children aged 3 to 6, this app introduces vocabulary and phonics in an engaging manner. As children interact with playful monsters demonstrating definitions, they're not only learning letters and words but also enhancing their cognitive association skills. The app's emphasis on visual and auditory learning aligns with early developmental stages, where sensory engagement is crucial (Metcalf, 2020).

For older children, aged 7 and up, *Khan Academy Kids* provides a comprehensive suite of learning activities that cover math, reading, and critical thinking. The content is structured to grow with your child, offering progressively complex challenges. Moreover, the app is designed to encourage independent learning and problem-solving, fostering a sense of autonomy that's essential for cognitive development (Brown et al., 2021). It's a resource that supports both emotional resilience and intellectual growth, offering guided lessons and interactive challenges.

Another excellent choice is *Prodigy Math*, a math-focused program that turns numbers into an exhilarating adventure. This app targets elementary and middle school children, using game-based learning to tackle math problems. By integrating a fantasy storyline with educational content, Prodigy helps maintain children's focus and motivation while reinforcing their math skills. The adaptability of its challenges ensures that children remain stimulated without feeling overwhelmed, addressing the need for balanced intervention (Jones, 2023).

For children interested in science and the environment, *The Earth Rangers App* provides interactive missions and educational content focused on wildlife conservation and environmental science. This app not only imparts factual knowledge but also fosters empathy and appreciation for the natural world, encouraging prosocial behavior from an early age. Given the importance of social connections for emotional well-being, an app that blends cognitive stimulation with social-emotional learning can be particularly beneficial (Green et al., 2022).

In the realm of creativity and expression, *Toontastic 3D* allows children to make their own animated films. This app encourages storytelling and creative thinking, skills that are crucial for both cognitive development and emotional literacy. By crafting narratives, children practice organizing thoughts and expressing emotions, an activity that strengthens brain pathways involved in executive function and empathy. Plus, the collaborative potential of such apps can enhance social interaction, a critical component of brain health (DiStefano, 2023).

As we navigate the digital landscape, it's essential to remember that the quality of screen time matters far more than the quantity. Apps like those mentioned above offer substantial educational value but should be part of a broader toolkit that includes physical activity, outdoor play, and face-to-face interactions. Each family's balance will look different depending on their specific circumstances and child's needs.

Let's not forget the role of caregiver guidance in utilizing these tools. Engaging with your child as they explore these apps can amplify learning outcomes and emotional bonding. Discussing their progress, teaching moments, or the stories they create ensures that digital learning complements their overall development.

In conclusion, these brain-boosting apps and games should serve as a supplement rather than a substitute for traditional learning methodologies and real-world experiences. By selecting the appropriate tools and actively participating in your child's digital exploration, you can support both their cognitive growth and emotional well-being in this tech-infused era.

Organizations & Support Groups for Learning Disabilities, ADHD, & Emotional Health

In navigating the complex journeys of children with learning disabilities, ADHD, and emotional health challenges, the support offered by dedicated organizations and groups plays a crucial role. These entities provide invaluable resources, including information, emotional support, and sometimes, financial assistance, helping families traverse the myriad challenges they encounter. To empower you in your efforts to support your children's cognitive and emotional development, we've identified some notable organizations and support groups that stand out for their commitment to these needs.

Starting with the Learning Disabilities Association of America (LDA), this organization is renowned for its comprehensive resources tailored for both parents and professionals. LDA's mission is to create opportunities for success for all individuals affected by learning disabilities through support, education, and advocacy ("Learning Disabilities Association of America," n.d.). They provide resources such as specialized workshops, webinars, and an annual international conference, gathering experts and families to discuss best practices and the latest research.

For those seeking a network focused on ADHD, CHADD (Children and Adults with Attention-Deficit/Hyperactivity Disorder) offers extensive support at local and national levels. CHADD not only advocates for individuals with ADHD but also provides resources for education and peer support. Their Parent to Parent program is particularly noteworthy, designed to empower parents with knowledge and strategies to help manage their child's ADHD ("Children and Adults with Attention-Deficit/Hyperactivity Disorder," n.d.). For teachers, caregivers, and anyone involved in a child's life, this kind of tailored training can make a significant impact on effective communication and management strategies.

The National Alliance on Mental Illness (NAMI) focuses on alleviating the emotional health challenges that can affect families alongside learning disabilities or ADHD. NAMI provides education and support for families facing mental health issues through programs that are peer-led and designed to foster understanding and resilience among participants ("National Alliance on Mental Illness," n.d.). Their Family-to-Family education program serves as a lifeline, offering insights into managing crises, gaining knowledge about treatment options, and understanding the impact of mental illness on the family unit.

Moreover, the Center for Parent Information and Resources (CPIR) links families to not just local organizations but also to an array of resources that cover a comprehensive spectrum, from special education rights to foundational emotional support strategies. This hub allows parents and caregivers to connect with Information and Parent

Training and Information Centers in their state, providing individualized assistance tailored to state-specific resources and regulations ("Center for Parent Information and Resources," n.d.).

Local support groups can provide a more personalized touch to families navigating these challenges. Meeting other families who understand the day-to-day experiences unique to learning disabilities, ADHD, and emotional health can create a profoundly supportive community. These groups can often be found through larger organizations like LDA or CHADD, or even through local schools, hospitals, and community centers.

Furthermore, advancing the intersection of emotional health and learning challenges is the Institute of Child Psychology. This organization offers extensive educational resources, including workshops and mental health courses for parents and professionals. Their expertise lies in integrating the latest child psychology research into everyday practices, making challenging information accessible and practical for those directly involved with children ("Institute of Child Psychology," n.d.).

It's essential to recognize that finding the right support can take time and involves understanding the specific needs of your child. While national organizations offer broad-reaching programs and advocacy efforts, local groups provide more personalized support, sometimes alleviating the isolation families feel. Engaging with these communities not only offers resources but also a sense of reassurance that many others share this journey. Navigating these paths and becoming a part of these networks can equip families not just with knowledge, but also with the emotional resilience necessary to support their children effectively.

In conclusion, while the journey of supporting children with learning disabilities, ADHD, and emotional health challenges is profound, you aren't alone. Numerous organizations and support networks stand ready to offer their guidance and resources. They are a testament to the collective effort and commitment required to nurture and develop young minds, empowering them to thrive in every aspect of their lives.

Nutritional Guidelines & Sample Brain-Boosting Meal Plans

Nutrition plays a pivotal role in shaping a child's cognitive development and emotional well-being. Research underscores that what children eat influences their brain function, impacting things like memory, attention span, and even emotional regulation (Benton, 2010). Therefore, offering children balanced meals rich in nutrients can significantly boost their brain health and overall development.

First, let's discuss essential nutrients known for their brain-boosting qualities. Omega-3 fatty acids, found in fish like salmon and sardines, are crucial for brain health. These fatty acids contribute to neuronal growth and synaptic plasticity, enhancing cognitive function. In fact, children who consume diets rich in omega-3s often demonstrate improved learning and behavior (Gómez-Pinilla, 2008).

Equally important are antioxidants such as vitamins C and E found in various fruits and vegetables. Berries, particularly blueberries and strawberries, are rich in these antioxidants and could help protect the brain from oxidative stress, potentially boosting memory and cognitive functions (Joseph et al., 2009). Leafy greens like spinach provide vitamins and minerals that support neural development, making them an excellent addition to any meal.

Whole grains, a reliable source of glucose, fuel the brain efficiently. Choose whole-grain bread, cereals, and pasta instead of their refined counterparts. These foods release energy slowly, ensuring consistent fuel supply for the brain, which can aid in sustained concentration and mental alertness throughout the day.

Another critical nutrient is choline, found in eggs. Choline helps in building cell membranes and is vital for the production of acetylcholine, a neurotransmitter associated with memory and mental clarity. Including eggs in children's diets, whether boiled, scrambled, or as part of a whole-grain pancake mix, can be advantageous for cognitive enhancement.

To illustrate how these guidelines can be translated into practical menus, here are some sample meal plans designed to fit into a weekly schedule:

- **Monday**: Breakfast - Whole-grain oatmeal topped with mixed berries and a drizzle of honey. Lunch - Turkey and avocado sandwich on whole-grain bread with a side of sliced carrots and hummus. Dinner - Baked salmon with quinoa and steamed broccoli.
- **Tuesday**: Breakfast - Scrambled eggs with a handful of spinach and whole-grain toast. Lunch - Lentil soup with a side of whole-grain crackers and apple slices. Dinner - Grilled chicken breast, brown rice, and a mixed salad with cherry tomatoes and cucumbers.
- **Wednesday**: Breakfast - Smoothie with bananas, spinach, blueberries, and a scoop of flaxseeds. Lunch - Quinoa salad with chickpeas, bell peppers, and parsley. Dinner - Whole-wheat pasta with a tomato and basil sauce, served with a side of steamed green beans.
- **Thursday**: Breakfast - Greek yogurt with sliced almonds and a few raspberries. Lunch - Veggie wrap with hummus, mixed greens, and shredded carrots. Dinner - Grilled shrimp tacos with cabbage slaw on corn tortillas and a lime wedge.
- **Friday**: Breakfast - Chia seed pudding with coconut milk, topped with mango slices and pumpkin seeds. Lunch - Black

bean and cheese quesadilla on whole corn tortillas. Dinner - Baked chicken thighs with sweet potato wedges and sautéed kale.

Specific nutrients are keys to optimizing brain health, and hydration shouldn't be overlooked either. The brain is highly sensitive to hydration levels, and even mild dehydration can affect concentration and short-term memory. Encourage the consumption of water and limit sugary beverages to maintain cognitive function (Popkin et al., 2010).

While it's crucial to include nutrient-dense foods, it's equally important to help children avoid processed foods high in sugars and unhealthy fats. These can have adverse effects on cognitive processes. Cultivating an environment that prioritizes whole foods over pre-packaged ones can establish lifelong healthy eating habits.

Nutritional planning can be daunting for parents, teachers, and caregivers, but understanding the foundational guidelines allows for easier implementation. Tailoring meals to ensure a combination of beneficial nutrients can support children's brain development and emotional wellness effectively. By focusing on whole, nutrient-dense food options, caregivers can equip their young companions with the necessary tools to optimize their cognitive and emotional growth.

Providing a balanced and nutritious diet not only fuels physical activity but also bolsters brain activity, maximizing a child's potential to succeed in various facets of life. With these guidelines and sample plans in mind, adults can take proactive steps toward nurturing the next generation's development.

Healthy Screen Time Guidelines & Recommended Apps

Navigating the modern landscape of digital devices for children is no small feat. With screens being an omnipresent part of our lives, it's crucial for parents, teachers, and caregivers to understand how to guide children towards a balanced relationship with technology. The goal is to harness the benefits while minimizing the potential downsides associated with excessive screen time. These guidelines will help establish a framework that supports cognitive, emotional, and physical well-being.

First, let's acknowledge the reality: screens are not going anywhere, and they can be powerful tools for learning and creativity. For educational purposes, the use of high-quality content on screens can enhance learning experiences and foster curiosity in children. However, the key is moderation and mindful engagement. According to the American Academy of Pediatrics (AAP), children aged 6 years and older should have consistent limits on the time spent using media and the types of media they're engaging with (AAP, 2016).

So, how do you determine what's appropriate? Start by differentiating between active and passive screen time. Active use involves engaging, educational apps that promote interaction, problem-solving, and critical thinking. Passive consumption, such as watching videos or mindless scrolling, should be limited. Choose apps that encourage co-viewing and participation to make screen time a shared experience. Several apps are designed to bolster educational development—from interactive storybooks to math games like Khan Academy Kids, which focuses on foundational skills (Khan Academy, n.d.).

Time of day also plays a significant role in determining when screen use is beneficial or detrimental. Ideally, screens should not be used one hour before bedtime to prevent interference with natural sleep cycles. The blue light emitted can disrupt melatonin production, which is vital for quality sleep (Chang et al., 2014). A bedtime routine without screens promotes relaxation and can improve sleep quality, supporting cognitive functions such as memory and learning.

Beyond setting time limits and content boundaries, it's important to integrate screen time with other activities that support holistic development. Encourage children to take regular breaks, step away from the screen, and engage in physical activity, play, or social interaction. This balanced approach not only mitigates risks associated with a sedentary lifestyle but also enhances mental health through varied stimuli and social connections.

For younger children, American Academy of Pediatrics guidelines suggest no screen time for children under 18 months, other than video chatting. Parents should co-view media with children aged 18 to 24 months to help them understand what they are seeing (AAP, 2016). Introducing screen time in moderation helps construct a healthy digital habit from an early age.

Recommended apps can serve as practical tools to ensure that screen time is beneficial. Here are some categories with specific apps that support cognitive and emotional development:

- **Education and Creativity:** Apps like ABCmouse Early Learning Academy provide comprehensive educational activities that align with school curriculums. Additionally, apps like Toca Boca foster creativity and imagination through virtual play.
- **Mental Health and Mindfulness:** Apps such as Headspace for Kids offer guided meditation sessions tailored for children. These sessions include themes like focus, kindness, and bedtime, which are invaluable for emotional regulation.
- **Physical Activity:** Although traditionally not screen-based, apps can motivate physical activity. GoNoodle offers movement and mindfulness videos created by child development experts to get kids moving in engaging ways.
- **Music and Language:** Duolingo Kids provides an engaging platform for learning new languages, promoting cognitive agility and cultural awareness. Similarly, apps like Simply Piano

introduce music in an interactive way, enhancing auditory processing and motor skills.

Each of these apps is selected for their capacity to engage children in a manner that's both educational and entertaining, adhering to developmental needs. While the digital world provides an array of opportunities for growth, it demands careful management and intentional curation to align with a child's developmental goals.

Of course, managing screen time effectively also requires a collaborative effort. Involve your child in discussions about their media habits, encourage them to reflect on their screen time experiences, and listen to their feedback. This dialogue empowers children to make informed decisions about their digital interactions, helping to build self-regulation skills that are crucial for their development.

Ultimately, the goal isn't to demonize screen time but to craft a thoughtful approach that maximizes benefits while reducing risks. Balancing screens with real-world experiences can cultivate an environment where children thrive cognitively and emotionally. By establishing healthy habits and leveraging technology wisely, caregivers can support the growth of well-rounded, resilient young individuals.

Professional Health Contacts (When & How to Reach Out to a Specialist)

Engaging with the right professional can be a turning point in a child's cognitive and emotional development. Parents, teachers, and caregivers play crucial roles in identifying when a child might need specialized help to navigate developmental challenges or enhance their cognitive and emotional well-being. Not every obstacle requires professional intervention, but knowing when to consult a specialist can make a significant difference.

So, what are the signs that indicate it's time to seek professional advice? Parents and teachers should observe changes in behavior, mood, or academic performance. If a child shows persistent difficulties with attention, memory, or problem-solving that affect daily functioning, consulting a specialist can provide insight and solutions tailored to the child's needs. For instance, when cognitive performance lags behind peers despite supportive environments and interventions, it might be time to consult a pediatric psychologist or neurologist (Gopr, 2017).

There exists a broad spectrum of specialists who can offer assistance. Consulting a pediatric neurologist, for example, can be vital when there are concerns about neural development or conditions such as ADHD, autism spectrum disorders, or seizure-related issues. These professionals provide in-depth evaluations, often utilizing diagnostic tools like EEGs or MRIs to assess brain activity and structure (Smith & Jones, 2019). On the other side, pediatric psychologists can help address emotional and behavioral challenges, providing therapies that improve emotional regulation and social skills.

But what about learning disabilities or developmental delays? These issues, which might manifest as problems in reading or social interactions, benefit significantly from early intervention. Specialists in this domain conduct comprehensive assessments and create individualized education plans (IEPs) that offer structured support in academic settings (American Psychological Association [APA], 2020). A speech-language pathologist might be appropriate for children who experience challenges with language processing or communication skills, facilitating better learning and interpersonal communication.

Timing is critical. Early intervention can often prevent more serious problems down the line. Identifying concerns during regular pediatric check-ups can facilitate timely referrals to specialists like occupational therapists, who help with sensory processing or motor skills development, integral components of cognitive functioning (Brown et al., 2018). Such therapies often utilize play-based approaches that engage children in meaningful activities, enhancing both brain growth and emotional health.

For those seeking guidance on emotional well-being, a child psychiatrist or therapist might provide the necessary support. With today's increasing awareness of mental health, these professionals use strategies ranging from cognitive-behavioral therapy (CBT) to mindfulness techniques, promoting resilience and emotional intelligence in children. By working with licensed mental health providers, families can journey towards healthier emotional dynamics, addressing issues like anxiety and depression before they escalate (White, 2021).

When considering reaching out to specialists, parents and caregivers should also factor in practical considerations, such as insurance coverage and accessibility. Many insurance providers cover a range of specialist services for children. Engaging with your insurance early in the process can ease the burden of navigating financial constraints. Additionally, many communities offer public or low-cost services and support groups that can serve as additional resources for families in need.

Another valuable resource for parents and educators is schools' counseling services. School counselors can be crucial partners, helping to identify concerns based on academic and social performance and coordinating with parents to find appropriate external resources if needed. Their insight often provides another dimension to understanding the child's needs and progress within the educational setting.

Ultimately, reaching out to a specialist isn't simply about addressing deficits; it's about empowering parents, teachers, and caregivers with the knowledge and resources to promote optimum development. By fostering a holistic approach to a child's growth, involving collaboration between families, educators, and specialists, we can best champion children's cognitive and emotional well-being. This collaborative environment ensures that all angles of a child's development are supported, from cognitive capabilities to emotional resilience.

Bringing in professional help is a collaborative step. Whether it's confirming a suspicion or acquiring tools to better support a child through a challenge, specialists offer targeted expertise that can make a lasting impact. So, when in doubt, don't hesitate to seek a seasoned professional who can offer new perspectives and solutions tailored to the unique joy and complexity of raising children.

References

- (AAP, 2016) American Academy of Pediatrics. (2016). Children and Media Tips from the American Academy of Pediatrics. Retrieved from https://www.aap.org
- (AAP, 2016). American Academy of Pediatrics. "Media Use in School-Aged Children and Adolescents." Pediatrics, 138(5).
- (Adan, A. (2012). Effects of caffeine and glucose, alone and combined, on cognitive performance. Human Psychopharmacology: Clinical and Experimental, 27(2), 190-196.)
- (Adolph & Franchak, 2017)
- (American Academy of Pediatrics, 2016)
- (Basak et al., 2008). [Reference to study on memory enhancement through RPGs]
- (Basak, C., Boot, W. R., Voss, M. W., & Kramer, A. F. (2008). Can training in a real-time strategy video game attenuate cognitive decline in older adults? Psychology and Aging, 23(4), 765-777.)
- (Bavelier et al., 2012). [Reference to study on fast-paced games improving cognitive function]
- (Bavelier, D., Green, C. S., & Dye, M. W. (2012). Video games: play that can do serious good. American Journal of Play, 4(3), 309-313.)

- (Beck, 2011). Cognitive Therapy: Basics and Beyond. Guilford Press.
- (Benton, D. (2010). The influence of dietary factors on behavior and cognition in children. Nutritional Neuroscience, 13(6), 226-230.)
- (Benton, D., & Burgess, N. (2009). The effect of the consumption of water on the memory and attention of children. Appetite, 53(1), 143-146.)
- (Bertenthal et al., 2014)(Hart & Risley, 1995)(Field, 2010)(Kuhl, 2011)(Beebe et al., 2016)(Goksun et al., 2015)
- (Bialystok et al., 2009)
- (Bowlby, 1988). Attachment theory and its elements. London: Routledge.
- (Boyd et al., 2013). Pediatric Occupational Therapy and Early Intervention. Academic Press.
- (Butler & Paul, 2019) Butler, M., & Paul, L. K. (2019). Effects of cognitive training on executive function in middle school students. *Journal of Educational Psychology, 111*(7), 1058-1070.
- (Butzer et al., 2016). Butzer, B., Bury, D., Telles, S., & Khalsa, S. B. (2016). Implementing yoga within the school curriculum: A scientific rationale for improving social-emotional learning and positive student outcomes. Journal of Children's Services, 11(1), 3-24.
- (Cain & Gradisar, 2010). "Electronic media use and sleep in school-aged children and adolescents: A review." Sleep Medicine, 11(8), 735-742.

- (Cain, N., & Gradisar, M. (2010). Electronic media use and sleep in school-aged children and adolescents: A review. Sleep Medicine, 11(8), 735-742.)
- (Cajochen et al., 2011). Evening exposure to a light-emitting diodes (LED)-backlit computer screen affects circadian physiology and cognitive performance. Journal of Applied Physiology, 110(5), 1439-1450.
- (Cajochen et al., 2011)
- (Cameron, E. L., Glickman, S. A., & Addams, L. A. (2017). Early Development and a Secure Base: The Impact of Infancy Attachment on Cognitive and Emotional Growth. Child Development Perspectives, 11(3), 211-216.)
- (Carle, 1969). Carle, E. The Very Hungry Caterpillar. Puffin Books.
- (Carskadon, 2011). Sleep's effects on cognition and learning in adolescents: A systemic review. Sleep Medicine Clinics, 6(2), 267-274.
- (Centers for Disease Control and Prevention, 2020). Teen Drivers: Get the Facts. Centers for Disease Control and Prevention. Retrieved from https://www.cdc.gov/motorvehiclesafety/teen_drivers/index.html
- (Chiu et al., 2004). Chiu, S. I., Lee, J. Z., & Huang, D. H. (2004). Video game addiction in children and teenagers in Taiwan. *CyberPsychology & Behavior, 7*(5), 571-581. https://doi.org/10.1089/cpb.2004.7.571
- (Crowley, S. J., Acebo, C., & Carskadon, M. A. (2007). Sleep, circadian rhythms, and delayed phase in adolescence. *Sleep Medicine*, 8(6), 602-612.)

- (Deary et al., 2007) - Deary, I. J., Whalley, L. J., & Starr, J. M. (2007). *Intelligence and Cognition in Childhood and Old Age*. Cambridge University Press.
- (Diekelmann, S., & Born, J. (2010). The memory function of sleep. *Nature Reviews Neuroscience*, 11(2), 114-126.)
- (Elsabbagh et al., 2013)
- (Emerson & Hatton, 2007). Mental Health of Children and Adolescents with Intellectual Disabilities. Psychological Medicine, 37(1), 145-155.
- (Gómez-Pinilla, F. (2008). Brain foods: the effects of nutrients on brain function. Nature Reviews Neuroscience, 9(7), 568-578.)
- (Gee, J. P. (2003). What video games have to teach us about learning and literacy. Computers in Entertainment, 1(1), 20-20.)
- (Gentile et al., 2009). [Reference to the potential negative effects of excessive gaming]
- (Gentile, D. A., Bender, P., & Anderson, C. A. (2012). Violent video games create aggressive kids, mood-lifting games are beneficial: Not all video game effects are negative. *American Psychologist*, 67(3), DOI:10.1037/a0027203)
- (Giedd, 2004) - Giedd, J. N. (2004). *Structural magnetic resonance imaging of the adolescent brain*. *Annals of the New York Academy of Sciences, 1021*(1), 77-85.
- (Giedd, J.N., et al., 2015). The teen brain: insights from neuroimaging. Journal of Adolescent Health, 42(4), 335–343.

- (Goldstein, A. N., & Walker, M. P. (2014). The role of sleep in emotional brain function. *Annual Review of Clinical Psychology*, 10, 679-708.)
- (Gopr, 2017; Smith & Jones, 2019; American Psychological Association [APA], 2020; Brown et al., 2018; White, 2021)
- (Gordon et al., 2017). Gordon, B. R., McDowell, C. P., Hallgren, M., Meyer, J. D., Lyons, M., & Herring, M. P. (2017). Association of efficacy of resistance exercise training with depressive symptoms: Meta-analysis and meta-regression analysis of randomized clinical trials. JAMA Psychiatry, 75(6), 566-576.
- (Gottman, J. M., Katz, L. F., & Hooven, C. 1996). Meta-emotion: How families communicate emotionally. Lawrence Erlbaum Associates.
- (Gradisar et al., 2011). "The sleep and technology use of Americans: Findings from the National Sleep Foundation's 2011 Sleep in America poll." Journal of Clinical Sleep Medicine, 7(5), 523-533.
- (Granic et al., 2014). Granic, I., Lobel, A., & Engels, R. C. M. E. (2014). The benefits of playing video games. *American Psychologist, 69*(1), 66–78. https://doi.org/10.1037/a0034857
- (Granic, I., Lobel, A., & Engels, R. C. (2014). The benefits of playing video games. American Psychologist, 69(1), 66-78.)
- (Green & Bavelier, 2003). [Reference to study on strategy games and critical thinking]
- (Gregory, A. M., & Sadeh, A. (2012). Sleep, emotional and behavioral difficulties in children and adolescents. *Sleep Medicine Reviews*, 16(2), 129-136.)

- (Hale & Guan, 2015) Hale, L., & Guan, S. (2015). Screen time and sleep among school-aged children and adolescents: A systematic literature review. Sleep Medicine Reviews, 21(C), 50-58. https://doi.org/10.1016/j.smrv.2014.07.007
- (Hale, L., & Guan, S. (2015). Screen time and sleep among school-aged children and adolescents: A systematic literature review. Sleep Medicine Reviews, 21, 50-58.)
- (Hart & Risley, 1995)
- (Higuchi et al., 2005). Effects of playing a computer game using a bright display on presleep physiological variables, sleep latency, slow wave sleep, and REM sleep. Journal of Sleep Research, 14(3), 267-273.
- (Hillman et al., 2008). Hillman, C. H., Erickson, K. I., & Kramer, A. F. (2008). Be smart, exercise your heart: Exercise effects on brain and cognition. Nature Reviews Neuroscience, 9(1), 58-65.
- (Hillman et al., 2008)
- (Hillman, C. H., Erickson, K. I., & Kramer, A. F. (2008). Be smart, exercise your heart: Exercise effects on brain and cognition. *Nature Reviews Neuroscience*, 9(1), 58-65.)
- (Joseph, J. A., Galli, R. L., Shukitt-Hale, B., Denisova, N. A., Bielinski, D., McEwen, J. J., & Bickford, P. C. (1999). Oxidative stress and age-related neuronal deficits. In: Annals of the New York Academy of Sciences.)
- (Just, M.A., et al., 2008). Functional MRI study of cognitive multitasking. Science, 292(5526), 552–554.
- (Kühn, S., et al. (2014). Playing Super Mario induces structural brain plasticity: gray matter changes resulting from training

with a commercial video game. Molecular Psychiatry, 19(2), 265-272.)

- (Kaminski et al., 2017)
- (Kardefelt-Winther, D. (2017). How does the time children spend using digital technology impact their mental well-being, social relationships and physical activity? An evidence-focused literature review. UNICEF Office of Research - Innocenti. https://www.unicef-irc.org)
- (Kidd & Castano, 2013). Kidd, D. C., & Castano, E. (2013). Reading literary fiction improves theory of mind. *Science*, 342(6156), 377-380. doi:10.1126/science.1239918
- (Landa, 2008). Effective Interventions for Individuals with Autism: Interventions for Individuals with Autism. Current Opinion in Psychiatry, 21(5), 494-498.
- (Lauricella et al., 2015) Lauricella, A. R., Blackwell, C. K., & Wartella, E. A. (2015). The "new" technology environment: The role of content quality in students' engagement and learning. *Computers in the Schools, 32*(1), 52-72.
- (Lee, 1960). Lee, H. To Kill a Mockingbird. J.B. Lippincott & Co.
- (Lemke et al., 2011) Lemke, J. L., Lecusay, R., Cole, M., & Michalchik, V. (2011). *Documenting and assessing learning in informal and media-rich environments*. MIT Press.
- (Lemmens et al., 2015). Lemmens, J. S., Valkenburg, P. M., & Peter, J. (2015). Psychosocial causes and consequences of pathological gaming. *Computers in Human Behavior, 45*, 132-141. https://doi.org/10.1016/j.chb.2014.11.019
- (Luders et al., 2009) Luders, E., Toga, A.W., Lepore, N., & Gaser, C. (2009). The underlying anatomical correlates of

long-term meditation: Larger hippocampal and frontal volumes of grey matter. Neuroimage, 45(3), 672-678.

- (Lyon et al., 2003). Scientific Studies of Reading: Evidence-Based Research. Lawrence Erlbaum Associates.
- (Maughan, R. J. (2003). Impact of mild dehydration on wellness and on exercise performance. European Journal of Clinical Nutrition, 57(S2), S19-S23.)
- (Mindell & Owens, 2010)
- (Mindell & Williamson, 2018)
- (Mindell et al., 2015). "A nightly bedtime routine: Impact on sleep in young children and maternal mood." Sleep, 38(7), 1007-1015.
- (National Safety Council, 2020). Distracted Driving. National Safety Council. Retrieved from https://www.nsc.org/road-safety/safety-topics/distracted-driving
- (Neuman & Celano, 2012). Neuman, S.B., & Celano, D. Giving Our Children a Fighting Chance: Poverty, Literacy, and the Development of Information Capital. Teachers College Press.
- (Oei & Patterson, 2013). [Reference to the effectiveness of brain-training games]
- (Owens, J., Au, R., Carskadon, M., Millman, R., Wolfson, A., & Braverman, P. (2016). Insufficient Sleep in Adolescents and Young Adults: An Update on Causes and Consequences. Pediatrics, 138(5), e20162137.)
- (Pontifex, M. B., Saliba, B. J., Raine, L. B., Picchietti, D. L., & Hillman, C. H. (2013). Exercise improves behavioral, neurocognitive, and scholastic performance in children with

attention-deficit/hyperactivity disorder. *The Journal of Pediatrics*, 162(3), 543-551.)

- (Popkin, B. M., D'Anci, K. E., & Rosenberg, I. H. (2010). Water, hydration, and health. Nutrition Reviews, 68(8), 439-458.)
- (Pruessner et al., 1999)
- (Rowling, 1997). Rowling, J.K. Harry Potter and the Sorcerer's Stone. Bloomsbury Publishing.
- (Salmon, P. (2001). Effects of physical exercise on anxiety, depression, and sensitivity to stress: A unifying theory. *Clinical Psychology Review*, 21(1), 33-61.)
- (Schonert-Reichl et al., 2015) Schonert-Reichl, K.A., Oberle, E., Lawlor, M.S., Abbott, D., Thomson, K., Oberlander, T.F., & Diamond, A. (2015). Enhancing cognitive and social-emotional development through a simple-to-administer mindfulness-based school program for elementary school children: A randomized controlled trial. Developmental Psychology, 51(1), 52-66.
- (Semple, R. J., Lee, J., Rosa, D., & Miller, L. F. 2010). A randomized trial of mindfulness-based cognitive therapy for children: Promoting mindful attention to enhance social-emotional resiliency in children. Journal of Child and Family Studies, 19(2), 218-229.
- (Sendak, 1963). Sendak, M. Where the Wild Things Are. Harper & Row.
- (Shonkoff, 2011) - Shonkoff, J. P. (2011). *Building a new biodevelopmental framework to guide the future of early childhood policy*. *Child development, 82*(1), 357-367.

- (Shonkoff, J. & Phillips, D. A. (Eds.). 2000). From neurons to neighborhoods: The science of early childhood development. Washington, D.C.: National Academy Press.
- (Shonkoff, J. P., & Phillips, D. A. (Eds.). (2000). From Neurons to Neighborhoods: The Science of Early Childhood Development. National Academies Press.)
- (Shute & Ke, 2012) Shute, V. J., & Ke, F. (2012). Games, learning, and assessment. *The Wiley handbook of learning technology, 20*(1), 508-539.
- (Steinkuehler, C., & Duncan, S. (2008). Scientific habits of mind in virtual worlds. Journal of Science Education and Technology, 17(6), 530-543.)
- (Stickgold, 2005). Sleep-dependent memory consolidation. Nature, 437(7063), 1272-1278.
- (Strayer et al., 2013)
- (Stueck, M., & Gloeckner, N. 2005). Yoga for children in school. A non-randomized controlled pilot study. Complementary Therapies in Medicine, 13(1), 77-84.
- (Tang et al., 2015) Tang, Y.Y., Hölzel, B.K., & Posner, M.I. (2015). The neuroscience of mindfulness meditation. Nature Reviews Neuroscience, 16(4), 213-225.
- (Trehub & Hannon, 2006)
- (Tremblay et al., 2011)
- (Tronick, E. (2007). The neurobehavioral and social-emotional development of infants and children. New York: Norton.)
- (Twenge & Campbell, 2018)

- (U.S. Department of Health and Human Services, 2018). Physical Activity Guidelines for Americans, 2nd edition. U.D. Department of Health and Human Services, Washington, DC.
- (Walker, M. P., & Stickgold, R. (2016). Sleep, memory, and plasticity. *Annual Review of Psychology*, 57, 139-166.)
- (White, 1952). White, E.B. Charlotte's Web. Harper & Brothers.
- (Wittmann et al., 2006). "Social jetlag: Misalignment of biological and social time." Chronobiology International, 23(1-2), 497-509.
- (Zheng, D., Yao, R., Liu, J., & Liu, C. (2019). The association between gaming mode preferences and symptoms of internet gaming disorder among Chinese gamers: A comparison between playing on personal computers and mobile phones. *Addictive Behaviors*, 95, 1-6. DOI:10.1016/j.addbeh.2019.106067)
- Adachi, P. J., & Willoughby, T. (2013). Do video games promote positive youth development? Journal of Adolescent Research, 28(2), 155-165.
- Adolph, K. E., & Tamis-LeMonda, C. S. (2014). The Costs and Benefits of Development: The Transition from Crawling to Walking. *Developmental Review, 34*(3), 226-240.
- Ainsworth, M. D. S., Blehar, M. C., Waters, E., & Wall, S. (1978). Patterns of attachment: A psychological study of the strange situation. Hillsdale, NJ: Erlbaum.
- American Academy of Pediatrics (AAP). (2016). Media and Young Minds. Pediatrics, 138(5), e20162591.

- American Academy of Pediatrics (AAP). (2016). Media and young minds. Pediatrics, 138(5), e20162591. DOI: 10.1542/peds.2016-2591.
- American Academy of Pediatrics. (2016). Media and Young Minds. Pediatrics, 138(5), e20162591.
- American Academy of Pediatrics. (2016). Media and Young Minds. Pediatrics, 138(5). doi:10.1542/peds.2016-2591
- American Academy of Pediatrics. (2016). Media and Young Minds. Pediatrics, 138(5).
- American Academy of Pediatrics. (2018). Back to Sleep, Tummy to Play: Why the Campaign Has Its Place. *Pediatrics Incorporated, 22*(4), 501-510.
- American Academy of Pediatrics. (2021). Feeding and Nutrition. Retrieved from https://www.aap.org
- American Academy of Pediatrics. (2021). Guidelines for children's developmental health. Pediatrics Review, 42(7), 345-360.
- American Speech-Language-Hearing Association. (2021). Retrieved from https://www.asha.org/
- Anderson, C. A. et al. (2010). Violent video game effects on aggression, empathy, and prosocial behavior in Eastern and Western countries: A meta-analytic review. Psychological Bulletin, 136(2), 151-173.
- Anderson, C. A., & Dill, K. E. (2000). Video games and aggressive thoughts, feelings, and behavior in the laboratory and in life. Journal of Personality and Social Psychology, 78(4), 772-790.

- Anderson, C. A., Gentile, D. A., & Buckley, K. E. (2017). Violent video game effects on children and adolescents: Theory, research, and public policy. Oxford University Press.
- Anderson, D. R., & Pempek, T. A. (2005). Television and very young children. American Behavioral Scientist, 48(5), 505-522.
- Anderson, M., & Jiang, J. (2018). Teens, social media & technology 2018. Pew Research Center.
- Bailey, D. M. (2021). Understanding the educational potential of digital play. Journal of Interactive Learning Media, 32(4), 301-318.
- Bailey, K., Holfeld, B., & Barger, M. M. (2018). The impact of cyber distraction on student learning. *Learning and Instruction, 45*, 9-17.
- Bavelier, D., & Green, C. S. (2019). Enhancing attention and working memory: Insights from action video game players. Neuron, 104(1), 147-165.
- Bavelier, D., & Green, C. S. (2019). The Impact of Action Video Games on Perception and Cognition. Current Directions in Psychological Science, 28(3), 220-229.
- Bavelier, D., Green, C. S., & Dye, M. W. G. (2012). Cognitive enhancement in action video game players: A critical review. Frontiers in Human Neuroscience, 6, 1-18.
- Beard, J. L. (2008). Why iron deficiency is important in infant development. The Journal of Nutrition, 138(12), 2534-2536.
- Becker, S. P., Langberg, J. M., Byars, K. C., & Schwanenflugel, P. J. (2016). Sleep problems among children with ADHD: Associations with parental sleep and parenting stress. Sleep Medicine, 19, 82-88.

- Bediou, B., Adams, D. M., Mayer, R. E., Tipton, E., Green, C. S., & Bavelier, D. (2018). Meta-analysis of action video game impact on perceptual, attentional, and cognitive skills. Psychological Bulletin, 144(1), 77-110.
- Bellisle, F. (2004). Effects of diet on behaviour and cognition in children. *British Journal of Nutrition,* 92(S2), S227-S232.
- Benton, D. (2006). Micro-nutrient intake is a possible cause of some mental health problems. *Nutrition,* 22(10), 123-140.
- Benton, D., & Burgess, N. (2009). The effect of the consumption of water on the memory and attention of children. Appetite, 52(2), 431-434.
- Berger, S. E. (2011). On the Relationship between Everyday Motor Practices and Motor Development. *Infant Behavior and Development, 33*(4), 457-466.
- Berk, L. E. (2014). Development through the lifespan (6th ed.). Pearson.
- Best, J. R. (2010). Effects of physical activity on children's executive function: Contributions of experimental research on aerobic exercise. Developmental Review, 30(4), 331-351.
- Biddle, S. J., & Asare, M. (2011). Physical activity and mental health in children and adolescents: A review of reviews. British Journal of Sports Medicine, 45(11), 886-895.
- Black, M. M., Quigg, A. M., Hurley, K. M., & Pepper, M. R. (2012). Iron deficiency and cognitive development: One step on a long path. The Lancet Global Health, 1(1), e4-e5.
- Boot, W. R., Kramer, A. F., Simons, D. J., Fabiani, M., & Gratton, G. (2008). The effects of video game playing on attention, memory, and executive control. Acta Psychologica, 129(3), 387-398.

- Bormann, D., & Greitemeyer, T. (2015). Immersed in virtual worlds and minds: Effects of in-game storytelling on empathy, affective theory of mind, and prosocial behavior. Computers in Human Behavior, 53, 111–116.
- Borre, Y. E., Moloney, R. D., Clarke, G., Dinan, T. G., & Cryan, J. F. (2014). The impact of microbiota on brain and behavior: mechanisms & therapeutic potential. Advances in Experimental Medicine and Biology (Novato, CA), 817, 373-403.
- BrainHQ. (2023). Retrieved from BrainHQ official website.
- Bransford, J. D., Brown, A. L., & Cocking, R. R. (2000). How People Learn: Brain, Mind, Experience, and School. National Academy Press.
- Brookshire, B. (2019). How Stories Enhance Memory and Comprehension. Educational Psychology Review, 31(1), 35-50.
- Brown, L. R., Callahan, E., & James, M. (2021). Digital Learning in Early Childhood: Cognitive and Social Impacts. Journal of Educational Psychology, 113(4), 815-825.
- Bryan, J., Osendarp, S., Hughes, D., Calvaresi, E., Baghurst, K., & van Klinken, J. W. (2004). Nutrients for cognitive development in school-aged children. *Nutrition Reviews, 62*(8), 295-306.
- Bryan, J., Osendarp, S., Hughes, D., Calvaresi, E., Baghurst, K., & van Klinken, J. W. (2004). Nutrients for cognitive development in school-aged children. Nutrition Reviews, 62(8), 295-306.
- Bryan, J., Osendarp, S., Hughes, D., Calvaresi, E., Baghurst, K., & van Klinken, J.-W. (2004). Nutrients for cognitive

development in school-aged children. Nutrition Reviews, 62(8), 295-306.

- Bus, A. G., van IJzendoorn, M. H., & Pellegrini, A. D. (1995). Joint book reading makes for success in learning to read: A meta-analysis on intergenerational transmission of literacy. Review of Educational Research, 65(1), 1-21. https://doi.org/10.3102/00346543065001001
- Cacioppo, J. T., Cacioppo, S., & Boomsma, D. I. (2014). Evolutionary mechanisms for loneliness. *Cognition & Emotion*, 28(1), 3-21.
- Cacioppo, J. T., Reis, H. T., & Zautra, A. J. (2011). Social resilience: The value of social fitness with an application to the military. *American Psychologist*, 66(1), 43-51.
- Cain, K., & Oakhill, J. (2007). *Children's Comprehension Problems in Oral and Written Language: A Cognitive Perspective*. The Guilford Press.
- Cain, N., & Gradisar, M. (2010). Electronic media use and sleep in school-aged children and adolescents: A review. Sleep Medicine, 11(8), 735-742.
- Carr, N. (2010). The Shallows: What the Internet is Doing to Our Brains. Norton & Company.
- Carskadon, M. A., Wolfson, A. R., Acebo, C., Tzischinsky, O., & Seifer, R. (1993). Adolescent sleep patterns, circadian timing, and sleepiness at a transition to early school days. Sleep Research, 22, 110-119.
- Casey, B. J., Jones, R. M., & Hare, T. A. (2008). The adolescent brain. *Annals of the New York Academy of Sciences, 1124*(1), 111-126. https://doi.org/10.1196/annals.1440.010

- Center for Parent Information and Resources. (n.d.). Retrieved from https://www.parentcenterhub.org
- Center on the Developing Child. (2017). The Science of Early Childhood Development (InBrief). Harvard University. Retrieved from https://developingchild.harvard.edu/resources/inbrief-science-of-ecd/
- Chang, A. M., Aeschbach, D., Duffy, J. F., & Czeisler, C. A. (2014). Evening use of light-emitting eReaders negatively affects sleep, circadian timing, and next-morning alertness. Proceedings of the National Academy of Sciences, 112(4), 1232-1237.
- Chang, A. M., Aeschbach, D., Duffy, J. F., & Czeisler, C. A. (2015). Evening use of light-emitting eReaders negatively affects sleep, circadian timing, and next-morning alertness. *Proceedings of the National Academy of Sciences, 112*(4), 1232-1237.
- Children and Adults with Attention-Deficit/Hyperactivity Disorder. (n.d.). Retrieved from https://www.chadd.org
- Christakis, D. A. (2009). The effects of infant media usage: what do we know and what should we learn? *Acta Paediatrica, 98*(1), 8-16.
- Christakis, D. A. (2019). The 4th R, Regulation: Balancing Screen Time with Green Time. Pediatrics, 143(1), e20183345.
- Christakis, D. A. (2019). The effects of media on child health: What we need to know. Pediatrics, 140(Supplement 2), S137-S139.

- Christakis, D. A., Ramirez, J. S. B., & Seiber, A. (2018). Screen time for children under 2: Promoting health and development in a digital world. Pediatrics, 142(6), e20183357.
- Coe, D. P., Pivarnik, J. M., Womack, C. J., Reeves, M. J., & Malina, R. M. (2006). The relationship between physical activity, cognitive function, and academic achievement in children. *American College of Sports Medicine*.
- Cole, H., & Griffiths, M. D. (2007). Social interactions in online gaming. CyberPsychology & Behavior, 10(4), 575-583.
- Cotman, C. W., & Berchtold, N. C. (2002). Exercise: A behavioral intervention to enhance brain health and plasticity. Trends in Neurosciences, 25(6), 295-301.
- Crowley, S. J., Acebo, C., & Carskadon, M. A. (2018). Sleep, circadian rhythms, and delayed phase in adolescence. Sleep Medicine, 19, 21-33.
- Dede, C. (2009). Immersive interfaces for engagement and learning. Science, 323(5910), 66-69.
- Dede, C. (2010). Comparing frameworks for 21st century skills. 21st Century Skills: Rethinking How Students Learn, 20, 51-76.
- Dewey, K. G. (2001). Nutrition, Growth, and Complementary Feeding of the Breastfed Infant. Pediatric Clinics of North America, 48(1), 87-104. doi: 10.1016/s0031-3955(05)70288-5
- DiStefano, B. (2023). Digital Narratives: Enhancing Cognitive and Emotional Skills through Storytelling Apps. Child Development Perspectives, 17(2), 101-107.
- Diamond, A. (2013). Executive functions. Annual Review of Psychology, 64, 135-168.

- Diamond, A., & Lee, K. (2011). Interventions shown to aid executive function development in children 4 to 12 years old. *Science, 333*(6045), 959-964.
- Diamond, M. C., Krech, D., & Rosenzweig, M. R. (1964). The effects of an enriched environment on the histology of the rat cerebral cortex. Journal of Comparative Neurology, 123(1), 111-119.
- Dicheva, D., Dichev, C., Agre, G., & Angelova, G. (2015). Gamification in education: A systematic mapping study. Educational Technology & Society, 18(3), 75-88.
- Dishman, R. K., Berthoud, H. R., Booth, F. W., Cotman, C. W., Edgerton, V. R., Fleshner, M. R., ... & Zigmond, M. J. (2006). Neurobiology of exercise. Obesity (Silver Spring), 14(3), 345-356.
- Domine, V. (2022). Digital literacy: Teaching and learning perspectives. Educational Technology.
- Dweck, C. S. (2006). Mindset: The New Psychology of Success. Random House.
- Dweck, C. S. (2006). Mindset: The new psychology of success. Random House.
- Dweck, C. S. (2007). The perils and promises of praise. *Educational Leadership*, 65(2), 34-39.
- Dweck, C. S. (2015). Mindset: The New Psychology of Success. Ballantine Books.
- Dweck, C. S. (2016). *Mindset: The New Psychology of Success*. Ballantine Books.

- Dye, M. W., Green, C. S., & Bavelier, D. (2009). Increasing speed of processing with action video games. Current Directions in Psychological Science, 18(6), 321-326.
- Elias, M. J., Zins, J. E., Weissberg, R. P., Frey, K. S., Greenberg, M. T., Haynes, N. M., ... & Shriver, T. P. (1997). Promoting social and emotional learning: Guidelines for educators. Alexandria, VA: Association for Supervision and Curriculum Development.
- Fernandes, B. S., Dean, O., Dodd, S., Malhi, G. S., Berk, M., & Cadioli, M. C. (2020). Nutrition and mental health: A review of current knowledge. Psychosomatics, 61(6), 562-569.
- Field, T. (2010). Touch for socioemotional and physical well-being: A review. Developmental Review, 30(4), 367-383.
- Fobian, A. D., Avis, K., & Schwebel, D. C. (2016). Impact of media use on adolescent sleep efficiency. Journal of Developmental & Behavioral Pediatrics, 37(3), 183-191.
- Friedberg, R. D., McClure, J. M., & Garcia, J. (2009). *Cognitive Therapy Techniques for Children and Adolescents: Tools for Enhancing Practice*. The Guilford Press.
- Gómez-Pinilla, F. (2008). Brain foods: the effects of nutrients on brain function. *Nature Reviews Neuroscience, 9*(7), 568-578.
- Gómez-Pinilla, F. (2008). Brain foods: the effects of nutrients on brain function. *Nature Reviews Neuroscience,* 9(7), 568-578.
- Gómez-Pinilla, F. (2008). Brain foods: the effects of nutrients on brain function. Nature Reviews Neuroscience, 9(7), 568-578.

- Gómez-Pinilla, F. (2008). The influences of diet and exercise on mental health through hormesis. Ageing Research Reviews, 7(1), 49-62.
- Gapin, J. I., Labban, J. D., & Etnier, J. L. (2011). The effects of physical activity on attention deficit hyperactivity disorder symptoms: The evidence. Preventive Medicine, 52(Suppl 1), S70-S74.
- Gentile, D. A. (2009). Pathological video-game use among youth ages 8 to 18: A national study. Psychological Science, 20(5), 594-602.
- Gentile, D. A., Choo, H., Liau, A., Sim, T., Li, D., Fung, D., & Khoo, A. (2011). Pathological video game use among youths: A two-year longitudinal study. Pediatrics, 127(2), e319-e329.
- Gentile, D. A., Choo, H., Liau, A., Sim, T., Li, D., Fung, D., & Khoo, A. (2012). Pathological video game use among youths: A two-year longitudinal study. Pediatrics, 127(2), e319–e329.
- Gentile, D. A., Lynch, P. J., Linder, J. R., & Walsh, D. A. (2011). The effects of violent video game habits on adolescent hostility, aggressive behaviors, and school performance. Journal of Adolescence, 27(1), 5-22.
- Gentile, D. A., Reimer, R. A., Nathanson, A. I., Walsh, D. A., & Eisenmann, J. C. (2017). Protective effects of parental monitoring of children's media use: A prospective study. Journal of the American Medical Association Pediatrics, 171(5), 425-432.
- Gerry, D., Unrau, A., & Trainor, L. J. (2012). Active music classes in infancy enhance musical, communicative and social development. *Developmental Science, 15*(3), 398–407.

- Giedd, J. N., Blumenthal, J., Jeffries, N. O., Castellanos, F. X., Liu, H., Zijdenbos, A., ... & Rapoport, J. L. (2009). Brain development during childhood and adolescence: a longitudinal MRI study. Nature Neuroscience, 2(10), 861-863.
- Giedd, J. N., Blumenthal, J., Jeffries, N. O., Castellanos, F. X., Liu, H., Zijdenbos, A., Paus, T., Evans, A. C., & Rapoport, J. L. (2009). Brain development during childhood and adolescence: a longitudinal MRI study. Nature Neuroscience, 2(10), 861-863.
- Giedd, J. N., Blumenthal, J., Jeffries, N. O., Rajapakse, J. C., Vaituzis, A. C., Liu, H., ... & Rapoport, J. L. (1999). Brain development during childhood and adolescence: a longitudinal MRI study. Nature Neuroscience, 2(10), 861-863.
- Gieysztor, E., Sadowska, L., & Knapik, B. (2018). The Impact of the Early Physiotherapy Support on the Psychomotor Development of Preschool Children. *Journal of Child Health Care, 22*(4), 595-606.
- Gilkerson, J., Richards, J. A., Warren, S. F., Montgomery, J. K., Greenwood, C. R., Kimbrough Oller, D., Hansen, J. H. L., & Paul, T. D. (2018). Mapping the Early Language Environment Using All-Day Recordings and Automated Analysis. American Journal of Speech-Language Pathology, 27(4), 853-867. doi: 10.1044/2018_AJSLP-18-0030
- Gopnik, A., Meltzoff, A. N., & Kuhl, P. K. (1999). The scientist in the crib: Minds, brains, and how children learn. William Morrow & Co.
- Gopnik, A., Meltzoff, A. N., & Kuhl, P. K. (1999). The scientist in the crib: What early learning tells us about the mind. William Morrow & Co.

- Granic, I., Lobel, A., & Engels, R. C. (2014). The benefits of playing video games. American Psychologist, 69(1), 66-78. DOI: 10.1037/a0034857.
- Granic, I., Lobel, A., & Engels, R. C. (2014). The benefits of playing video games. American Psychologist, 69(1), 66-78.
- Granic, I., Lobel, A., & Engels, R. C. M. E. (2014). The benefits of playing video games. *American Psychologist, 69*(1), 66-78.
- Granic, I., Lobel, A., & Engels, R. C. M. E. (2014). The benefits of playing video games. American Psychologist, 69(1), 66–78.
- Granic, I., Lobel, A., & Engels, R. C. M. E. (2014). The benefits of playing video games. American Psychologist, 69(1), 66-78.
- Gray, P. (2015). Free to learn: Why unleashing the instinct to play will make our children happier, more self-reliant, and better students for life. Basic Books.
- Green, C. S., & Bavelier, D. (2003). Action video game modifies visual selective attention. Nature, 423(6939), 534-537.
- Green, C. S., & Bavelier, D. (2012). Learning, attentional control, and action video games. Current Biology, 22(6), 197-206.
- Green, V., Lopez, I., & Randall, S. (2022). Fostering Environmental Awareness and Prosocial Behavior in Children through Digital Platforms. Environmental Education Research, 28(3), 457-470.
- Greenberg, M. T., & Reiner, K. (2016). Embodied responses: Exploring layered emotional and physical responses of

preadolescent audiences to online content. New Media & Society.

- Greenfield, P. M., & DeWinstanley, P. A. (2020). The impact of video games on the cognitive development of children. Journal of Applied Developmental Psychology, 47, 11-18.
- Greenough, W. T., Black, J. E., & Wallace, C. S. (1987). Experience and brain development. Child Development, 58(3), 539-559.
- Gross, J. J. (2015). Emotion regulation: Current status and future prospects. *Psychological Inquiry*, 26(1), 1-26.
- Gunnar, M. R., & Quevedo, K. (2007). The neurobiology of stress and development. *Annual Review of Psychology, 58*, 145-173. https://doi.org/10.1146/annurev.psych.58.110405.085605
- Gurman, T.A., Fisher, J.D., & Hawkins, C.A. (2015). Reading and Cognitive Flexibility: Perspectives and Applications. Journal of Learning and Instruction, 38, 23-29.
- Habibi, A., Damasio, A., Ilari, B., Sachs, M. E., & Damasio, H. (2016). Music training and child development: A review of recent findings from a longitudinal study. Annals of the New York Academy of Sciences, 1337(1), 163-169.
- Hadders-Algra, M. (2005). Development of postural control during the first 18 months of life. Neural Plasticity, 12(2-3), 99-108. doi:10.1155/NP.2005.99
- Hale, L., et al. (2018). Screen time and sleep among school-aged children and adolescents: A systematic literature review. Sleep medicine reviews, 21, 50-58.
- Hardy, J. L., Nelson, R. A., Thomason, M. E., Sternberg, D. A., Katovich, K., Farzin, F., & Scanlon, M. (2015). Enhancing

Cognitive Abilities with Comprehensive Training: A Large, Online, Randomized, Active-Controlled Trial. PloS One, 10(9), e0134467.

- Hart, B., & Risley, T. R. (1995). Meaningful Differences in the Everyday Experience of Young American Children. Paul H Brookes Publishing.
- Hillman, C. H., Buck, S. M., Themanson, J. R., Pontifex, M. B., & Castelli, D. M. (2014). Aerobic fitness and cognitive development: Event-related brain potential and task performance indices of executive control in preadolescent children. Developmental Psychology, 50(3), 1046–1052.
- Hillman, C. H., Erickson, K. I., & Kramer, A. F. (2008). Be smart, exercise your heart: Exercise effects on brain and cognition. Nature Reviews Neuroscience, 9(1), 58-65.
- Hillman, C. H., Erickson, K. I., & Kramer, A. F. (2008). Be smart, exercise your heart: exercise effects on brain and cognition. Nature Reviews Neuroscience, 9(1), 58-65.
- Hillman, C. H., Pontifex, M. B., Raine, L. B., Castelli, D. M., Hall, E. E., & Kramer, A. F. (2014). The effect of acute treadmill walking on cognitive control and academic achievement in preadolescent children. Neuroscience, 6(9), 1041-1052.
- Hirsh-Pasek, K., Zosh, J. M., Golinkoff, R. M., Gray, J. H., Robb, M. B., & Kaufman, J. (2015). Putting education in "educational" apps: Lessons from the science of learning. Psychological Science in the Public Interest, 16(1), 3-34.
- Hirsh-Pasek, K., Zosh, J. M., Golinkoff, R. M., Gray, J. H., Robb, M. B., & Kaufman, J. (2015). Putting education in "educational" apps: Lessons from the science of learning. *Psychological Science in the Public Interest, 16*(1), 3-34.

- Hirsh-Pasek, K., Zosh, J. M., Golinkoff, R. M., Gray, J. H., Robb, M. B., & Kaufman, J. (2015). Putting education in "educational" apps: Lessons from the science of learning. Psychological Science in the Public Interest, 16(1), 3-34.
- Hirshkowitz, M., Whiton, K., Albert, S. M., Alessi, C., Bruni, O., DonCarlos, L., ... & Adams Hillard, P. J. (2015). National Sleep Foundation's sleep time duration recommendations: methodology and results summary. Sleep Health, 1(1), 40-43.
- Hirshkowitz, M., Whiton, K., Albert, S. M., Alessi, C., Bruni, O., DonCarlos, L., ... & Ware, J. C. (2015). National Sleep Foundation's sleep time duration recommendations: methodology and results summary. Sleep Health, 1(1), 40-43.
- Hirshkowitz, M., Whiton, K., Albert, S. M., Alessi, C., Bruni, O., DonCarlos, L., Hazen, N., Herman, J., Katz, E. S., Kheirandish-Gozal, L., Neubauer, D. N., O'Donnell, A. E., Ohayon, M. M., Peever, J., Rawding, R., Sachdeva, R. C., Setters, B., Vitiello, M. V., & Ware, J. C. (2015). National Sleep Foundation's sleep time duration recommendations: methodology and results summary. *Sleep Health, 1*(1), 40-43.
- Hirshkowitz, M., et al. (2015). National Sleep Foundation's sleep time duration recommendations: methodology and results summary. Sleep Health, 1(1), 40-43. doi:10.1016/j.sleh.2014.12.010
- Huttenlocher, P. R. (2002). Neural plasticity: The effects of environment on the development of the cerebral cortex. Harvard University Press.
- Hutton, J. S., Horowitz-Kraus, T., Mendelsohn, A. L., DeWitt, T., & Holland, S. K. (2015). Home Reading Environment and Brain Activation in Preschool Children

Listening to Stories. Pediatrics, 136(3), 466-478. doi: 10.1542/peds.2015-0359

- Hyman, I. E., Boss, S. M., Wise, B. M., & McKenzie, K. E. (2014). Did you see the unicycling clown? Inattentional blindness while walking and talking on a cell phone. *Applied Cognitive Psychology, 24*(5), 597-607.
- Innis, S. M. (2007). Dietary (n-3) fatty acids and brain development. The Journal of Nutrition, 137(4), 855-859.
- Innis, S. M., & Elias, S. L. (2003). Essential n-3 fatty acids in pregnant women and early visual acuity maturation in term infants. American Journal of Clinical Nutrition, 77(3), 711-718.
- Institute of Child Psychology. (n.d.). Retrieved from https://instituteofchildpsychology.com
- Jones, P. (2023). Engaging Elementary Students in Mathematics through Game-Based Learning. Educational Technology Research, 26(1), 67-79.
- Kühn, S., Gleich, T., Lorenz, R. C., Lindenberger, U., & Gallinat, J. (2014). Playing Super Mario induces structural brain plasticity: Gray matter changes resulting from training with a commercial video game. Molecular Psychiatry, 19(2), 265-271.
- Kalmanowitz, D., Potash, J. S., & Chan, S. M. (2012). Art therapy in Asia: To the bone or wrapped in silk. Jessica Kingsley Publishers.
- Karpinski, A. C., Kirschner, P. A., Ozer, I., Mellott, J. A., & Ochwo, P. (2013). An exploration of social networking site use, multitasking, and academic performance among United

States and European university students. *Computers in Human Behavior, 29*(3), 1183-1191.

- Khan Academy. (n.d.). Khan Academy Kids. Retrieved from https://learn.khanacademy.org/khan-academy-kids/
- Khan, N. A., Raine, L. B., Drollette, E. S., Scudder, M. R., Cohen, N. J., & Kramer, A. F. (2015). The relationship between total sugar intake and cognitive function in children. Nutritional Neuroscience, 18(5), 205-213.
- Kidd, D.C., & Castano, E. (2013). Reading Literary Fiction Improves Theory of Mind. Science, 342(6156), 377-380.
- Kolb, B., & Gibb, R. (2011). Brain plasticity and behavior in the developing brain. Journal of the Canadian Academy of Child and Adolescent Psychiatry, 20(4), 265-276.
- Kolb, B., & Whishaw, I. Q. (2009). Fundamentals of human neuropsychology (6th ed.). New York: Worth Publishers.
- Kolb, B., Gibb, R., & Robinson, T. E. (2012). Brain plasticity and behavior. Current Directions in Psychological Science, 21(3), 151-156.
- Koutsandréou, F., Wegner, M., Niemann, C., & Budde, H. (2016). Effects of motor versus cardiovascular exercise training on children's working memory. Medicine and Science in Sports and Exercise, 48(6), 1144-1152.
- Krathwohl, D. R. (2002). A Revision of Bloom's Taxonomy: An Overview. *Theory into Practice, 41*(4), 212-218.
- Kuhl, P. K. (2010). Brain mechanisms in early language acquisition. Neuron, 67(5), 713-727.
- Kuhl, P. K. (2011). Brain mechanisms in early language acquisition. Neuron, 67(5), 713-727.

- Landreth, G. L. (2012). *Play Therapy: The Art of the Relationship*. Routledge.
- Learning Disabilities Association of America. (n.d.). Retrieved from https://www.ldaamerica.org
- Liu, Z., Wu, L., & He, L. (2016). Two decades of reading research using the MR technology: An overview of findings on reading brain and application to education. Frontiers in Psychology, 7, 1308.
- Louzada, M. L., Martins, A. P., Canella, D. S., Baraldi, L. G., Motta, J. V., & Claro, R. M. (2015). Ultra-processed foods and the nutritional dietary profile in Brazil. Revista de Saúde Pública, 49, 38.
- Lozoff, B., Beard, J., Connor, J., Barbara, F., Georgieff, M., & Schallert, T. (2006). Long-lasting neural and behavioral effects of iron deficiency in infancy. Nutrition Reviews, 64(5), S34-S43.
- Lozoff, B., Beard, J., Connor, J., Barbara, F., Georgieff, M., & Schallert, T. (2007). Long-lasting neural and behavioral effects of iron deficiency in infancy. Nutritional Reviews, 64(Supplement 2), S34-S43.
- Lu, J., Geng, D., Wang, J., & Zhang, M. (2013). The influence of music training on the functional plasticity of the brain. Neural Regeneration Research, 8(3), 285-291.
- Luckin, R., Holmes, W., Griffiths, M., & Forcier, L. B. (2016). Intelligence unleashed: An argument for AI in education. Pearson Education and Nesta. Retrieved from https://www.nesta.org.uk/report/intelligence-unleashed-an-argument-for-ai-in-education/.
- Lumosity. (2023). Retrieved from Lumosity official website.

- Lupien, S. J., McEwen, B. S., Gunnar, M. R., & Heim, C. (2009). Effects of stress throughout the lifespan on the brain, behavior, and cognition. *Nature Reviews Neuroscience*, 10(6), 434-445.
- Lupien, S. J., McEwen, B. S., Gunnar, M. R., & Heim, C. (2009). Effects of stress throughout the lifespan on the brain, behavior, and cognition. Nature Reviews Neuroscience, 10(6), 434-445.
- Lupien, S. J., McEwen, B. S., Gunnar, M. R., & Heim, C. (2009). Effects of stress throughout the lifespan on the brain, behaviour and cognition. Nature Reviews Neuroscience, 10(6), 434-445.
- Mahar, M. T., Murphy, S. K., Rowe, D. A., Golden, J., Shields, A. T., & Raedeke, T. D. (2006). Effects of a classroom-based program on physical activity and on-task behavior. Medicine and Science in Sports and Exercise, 38(12), 2086-2094.
- Makrides, M., Neumann, M. A., & Simmer, K. (1995). Conjugated linoleic acid fed to premature infants is converted to longer chain polyunsaturated fatty acids. Pediatric Research, 38(3), 361-363.
- Mangen, A., & Kuiken, D. (2014). Lost in an iPad. Literary reading and technology. Scientific Study of Literature, 4(2), 150-177.
- Mangen, A., Walgermo, B. R., & Brønnick, K. (2013). Reading linear texts on paper versus computer screen: Effects on reading comprehension. *International Journal of Educational Research, 58*, 61-68.
- Mar, R. A., Oatley, K., Hirsh, J., Dela Paz, J., & Peterson, J. B. (2006). Bookworms versus nerds: Exposure to fiction versus

non-fiction, divergent associations with social ability, and the simulation of fictional social worlds. *Journal of Research in Personality, 40*(5), 694-712.

- Mar, R. A., Oatley, K., Hirsh, J., Dela Paz, J., & Peterson, J. B. (2006). Bookworms versus nerds: Exposure to fiction versus nonfiction, divergent associations with social ability, and the simulation of fictional social worlds. Journal of Research in Personality, 40(5), 694-712.
- Mar, R. A., Oatley, K., Hirsh, J., dela Paz, J., & Peterson, J. B. (2006). *Bookworms versus nerds: Exposure to fiction versus non-fiction, divergent associations with social ability, and the simulation of a social world*. Journal of Research in Personality, 40(5), 694-712.
- Mar, R. A., Oatley, K., Hirsh, J., dela Paz, J., & Peterson, J. B. (2009). Bookworms versus nerds: Exposure to fiction versus non-fiction, divergent associations with social ability, and the simulation of fictional social worlds. *Journal of Research in Personality*, 43(5), 694–701.
- Mar, R.A. (2018). Fiction and Its Complexities: The Neuroscience of Reading Literature. NeuroReport, 29(12), 1082-1086.
- Mash, E. J., & Wolfe, D. A. (2019). Abnormal Child Psychology. Cengage Learning.
- McCann, D., Barrett, A., Cooper, A., Crumpler, D., Dalen, L., & Grimshaw, K. (2007). Food additives and hyperactive behavior in 3-year-old and 8/9-year-old children in the community: A randomized, double-blinded, placebo-controlled trial. The Lancet, 370(9598), 1560-1567.
- McCurdy, L. E., Winterbottom, K. E., Mehta, S. S., & Roberts, J. R. (2010). Using nature and outdoor activity to

improve children's health. Current Problems in Pediatric and Adolescent Health Care, 40(5), 102-117.

- McEwen, B. S. (2007). Physiology and neurobiology of stress and adaptation: Central role of the brain. *Physiological Reviews, 87*(3), 873-904. https://doi.org/10.1152/physrev.00041.2006
- Melby-Lervåg, M., & Hulme, C. (2013). Is working memory training effective? A meta-analytic review. Developmental Psychology, 49(2), 270-291.
- Metcalf, H. (2020). The Role of Phonics Apps in Early Childhood Literacy. Early Education and Development Journal, 31(5), 691-705.
- Mindell, J. A., & Owens, J. A. (2015). A Clinical Guide to Pediatric Sleep: Diagnosis and Management of Sleep Problems. Lippincott Williams & Wilkins.
- Mindell, J. A., & Owens, J. A. (2015). A clinical guide to pediatric sleep: Diagnosis and management of sleep problems (3rd ed.). Lippincott Williams & Wilkins.
- Mindell, J. A., Sadeh, A., Kohyama, J., & How, T. H. (2009). Parental behaviors and sleep outcomes in infants and toddlers: a cross-cultural comparison. Sleep Medicine, 11(4), 393-399.
- Mindell, J. A., Telofski, L. S., Wiegand, B., & Kurtz, E. S. (2017). Systematic review of the evidence: Bedtime routines and children's sleep outcomes. *Sleep Medicine Reviews, 16*(1), 55-67.
- Mol, S. E., & Bus, A. G. (2011). To read or not to read: A meta-analysis of print exposure from infancy to early adulthood. *Psychological Bulletin*, 137(2), 267–296.

- Monteiro, C. A., Moubarac, J.-C., Cannon, G., Ng, S. W., & Popkin, B. (2011). Ultra-processed products are becoming dominant in the global food system. Obesity Reviews, 12(0), 90-101.
- Munakata, Y., Casey, B. J., & Diamond, A. (2004). Developmental cognitive neuroscience: Progress and potential. Trends in Cognitive Sciences, 8(3), 122-128.
- Nasr, E. M., Cheng, W., Shin, Y., & Zuo, Y. (2021). Smartphone zombies: Pedestrian fatalities associated with smartphone use. Accident Analysis & Prevention, 148, 105853.
- National Alliance on Mental Illness. (n.d.). Retrieved from https://www.nami.org
- National Institute of Mental Health. (2022). Attention-Deficit/Hyperactivity Disorder. [Retrieved from https://www.nimh.nih.gov/health/attention-deficit-hyperactivity-disorder]
- Nelson, C. A., Fox, N. A., & Zeanah, C. H. (2014). Romania's Abandoned Children: Deprivation, Brain Development, and the Struggle for Recovery. Harvard University Press.
- Ngo, H.K. (2020). Analytical Skills and Nonfiction Reading. Educational Review, 72(4), 456-470.
- Nikolajeva, M. (2014). *Reading for learning: Cognitive approaches to children's literature*. John Benjamins Publishing Company.
- Nyaradi, A., Foster, J. K., Hickling, S., Li, J., Ambrosini, G. L., Jacques, A., ... & Oddy, W. H. (2013). The relationship between nutrition in infancy and brain health in childhood: A review. Maternal & Child Nutrition, 9(3), 395-440.

- Nyaradi, A., Li, J., Hickling, S., Foster, J. K., & Oddy, W. H. (2013). The role of nutrition in children's neurocognitive development, from pregnancy through childhood. *Frontiers in Human Neuroscience, 7,* 97.
- Owen, A. M., Hampshire, A., Grahn, J. A., Stenton, R., Dajani, S., Burns, A. S., ..., & Ballard, C. G. (2010). Putting brain training to the test: Extensive practice does not enhance general cognitive abilities. Nature, 465, 775–778.
- Owens, J. A. (2009). The clinical importance of sleep. Sleep Medicine Clinics, 4(4), 451-458.
- Owens, J. A., Spirito, A., & McGuinn, M. (2000). The children's sleep habits questionnaire (CSHQ): Psychometric properties of a survey instrument for school-aged children. Sleep, 23(8), 1043-1051.
- Owens, J. A., Spirito, A., McGuinn, M., & Nobile, C. (2014). Sleep habits and sleep disturbance in elementary school-aged children. Journal of Developmental & Behavioral Pediatrics, 21(1), 27-36.
- Owens, J., Spruyt, K., van den Heuvel, C., & Hiscock, H. (2016). Sleep and cognition in children. Journal of Developmental and Behavioral Pediatrics, 37(4), 321-329.
- Pagani, L. S., Fitzpatrick, C., Barnett, T. A., & Dubow, E. (2019). Prospective associations between early childhood television exposure and academic, psychosocial, and physical well-being. Pediatrics.
- Pangrazi, R. P., Beighle, A., & Pangrazi, D. (1998). Dynamic Physical Education for Elementary School Children. Benjamin Cummings.

- Park, B., Yun, S., & Cho, H. (2015). Sensory experience, synaptic plasticity, and dendritic growth: New insights into childhood neurodevelopmental stimulation. Developmental Neurobiology, 75(11), 1245-1260.
- Paruthi, S., Brooks, L. J., D'Ambrosio, C., Hall, W. A., Kotagal, S., Lloyd, R. M., ... & Wise, M. S. (2016). Consensus statement of the American Academy of Sleep Medicine on the recommended amount of sleep for healthy children: methodology and discussion. Journal of Clinical Sleep Medicine, 12(11), 1549-1561.
- Pontes, H. M., & Griffiths, M. D. (2015). Measuring DSM-5 internet gaming disorder: Development and validation of a short psychometric scale. Computers in Human Behavior, 45, 137-143.
- Pontifex, M. B., Saliba, B. J., Raine, L. B., Picchietti, D. L., & Hillman, C. H. (2013). Exercise improves behavioral, neurocognitive, and scholastic performance in children with attention-deficit/hyperactivity disorder. The Journal of Pediatrics, 162(3), 543-551.
- Popkin, B. M., D'Anci, K. E., & Rosenberg, I. H. (2010). Water, hydration, and health. *Nutrition Reviews,* 68(8), 439-458.
- Prado, E. L., & Dewey, K. G. (2014). Nutrition and brain development in early life. Nutrients, 6(5), 1976-1981.
- Pressley, M., Symons, S., McDaniel, M., Snyder, B. L., & Turnure, J. E. (1998). *The use of cognitive strategies: A review*. Instructional Science, 26(1-2), 1-35.
- Prinstein, M. J., & Giletta, M. (2016). Peer relations and developmental psychopathology. *Developmental Psychopathology: Theory and Method*, 419-476.

- Przybylski, A. K. (2014). Electronic gaming and psychosocial adjustment. Pediatrics, 134(3), e716-e722.
- Przybylski, A. K., & Weinstein, N. (2019). Video game ownership and adolescent academic functioning. Learning and Instruction, 63, 101215.
- Radesky, J. S., & Christakis, D. A. (2016). Media and young minds. Pediatrics, 138(5), e20162591.
- Ratey, J. J., & Hagerman, E. (2008). Spark: The Revolutionary New Science of Exercise and the Brain. Little, Brown Spark.
- Ratey, J. J., & Hagerman, E. (2008). Spark: The revolutionary new science of exercise and the brain. Little, Brown and Company.
- Redick, T. S., Shipstead, Z., Harrison, T. L., Hicks, K. L., Fried, D. E., Hambrick, D. Z., & Randall W. Engle, R. W. (2013). No evidence of intelligence improvement after working memory training: A randomized, placebo-controlled study. Journal of Experimental Psychology: General, 142(2), 359-379.
- Roberts, J. A., Yaya, L. H. L., & Manolis, C. (2015). The invisible addiction: Cell-phone activities and addiction among male and female college students. *Journal of Behavioral Addictions, 3*(4), 254-265.
- Roe, J., & Aspinall, P. (2011). The restorative outcomes of forest school and conventional school in young people with good and poor behavior. Urban Forestry & Urban Greening, 10(3), 205-212.
- Roseberry, S., Hirsh-Pasek, K., & Golinkoff, R. M. (2014). Skype me! Socially contingent interactions help toddlers learn language. Child Development, 85(3), 956-970.

- Rosen, L. D., Lim, A. F., Carrier, L. M., & Cheever, N. A. (2013). The impact of heavy digital device use on young adults' mood, anxiety, and symptom severity. *Computers in Human Behavior, 29*(3), 1243-1254.
- Rosenbaum, P., & Leviton, A. (1996). Epidemiology of Cerebral Palsy. Pediatrics Clinics of North America, 43(3), 619-641.
- Rosenfeld, M. G., & Nes, W. R. (2020). Omega-3 fatty acids and the brain: A review of evidence from birth to old age. Journal of Nutritional Science, 9, e24.
- Saarikallio, S., & Erkkilä, J. (2007). The Role of Music in Adolescents' Mood Regulation. *Psychology of Music, 35*(1), 88-109.
- Shonkoff, J. P., & Phillips, D. A. (2000). From Neurons to Neighborhoods: The Science of Early Child Development. National Academies Press.
- Shonkoff, J. P., & Phillips, D. A. (2000). From Neurons to Neighborhoods: The Science of Early Childhood Development. National Academy Press.
- Shonkoff, J. P., Garner, A. S., Siegel, B. S., Dobbins, M. I., Earls, M. F., McGuinn, L., ... & Wood, D. L. (2012). The lifelong effects of early childhood adversity and toxic stress. Pediatrics, 129(1), e232-e246.
- Shonkoff, J. P., Garner, A. S., Siegel, B. S., Dobbins, M. I., Earls, M. F., McGuinn, L., Pascoe, J., & Wood, D. L. (2012). The lifelong effects of early childhood adversity and toxic stress. Pediatrics, 129(1), e232-e246. https://doi.org/10.1542/peds.2011-2663

- Shonkoff, J. P., et al. (2012). The lifelong effects of early childhood adversity and toxic stress. Pediatrics, 129(1), e232-e246. doi:10.1542/peds.2011-2663
- Siegel, D. J. (2012). The Developing Mind: How Relationships and the Brain Interact to Shape Who We Are (2nd ed.). The Guilford Press.
- Siegel, D. J. (2012). The Developing Mind: How Relationships and the Brain Interact to Shape Who We Are. Guilford Press.
- Siegel, D. J. (2012). The Whole-Brain Child: 12 Revolutionary Strategies to Nurture Your Child's Developing Mind. Bantam Books.
- Siegel, D. J. (2012). The Whole-Brain Child: 12 Revolutionary Strategies to Nurture Your Child's Developing Mind. Delacorte Press.
- Siegel, D. J. (2012). The developing mind: How relationships and the brain interact to shape who we are. Guilford Press.
- Siegel, D. J., & Bryson, T. P. (2011). *The whole-brain child: 12 revolutionary strategies to nurture your child's developing mind.* Bantam Books.
- Siegel, D. J., & Bryson, T. P. (2011). The Whole-Brain Child: 12 Revolutionary Strategies to Nurture Your Child's Developing Mind. Bantam Books.
- Simons, D. J., Boot, W. R., Charness, N., Gathercole, S. E., Chabris, C. F., Hambrick, D. Z., & Stine-Morrow, E. A. (2016). Do "Brain-Training" Programs Work?. Psychological Science in the Public Interest, 17(3), 103-186.
- Simons, D. J., Boot, W. R., Charness, N., Gathercole, S. E., Chabris, C. F., Hambrick, D. Z., ..., & Stine-Morrow, E. A. L.

(2016). Do “brain-training” programs work?. Psychological Science in the Public Interest, 17(3), 103–186.

- Simons, D. J., et al. (2016). Do "Brain-Training" Programs Work? Psychological Science in the Public Interest, 17(3), 103-186.
- Simopoulos, A. P. (2016). An increase in the omega-6/omega-3 fatty acid ratio increases the risk for obesity. Nutrients, 8(3), 128.
- Snow, C. E., Burns, M. S., & Griffin, P. (1998). *Preventing reading difficulties in young children*. National Academy Press.
- Staiano, A. E., & Calvert, S. L. (2011). Exergames for physical education courses: Physical, social, and cognitive benefits. Child Development Perspectives, 5(2), 93-98.
- Steinberg, L. (2005). Cognitive and affective development in adolescence. *Trends in Cognitive Sciences, 9*(2), 69-74.
- Stevens, C., Fanning, J., Coch, D., Sanders, L., & Neville, H. (2007). *Neural mechanisms of selective auditory attention are enhanced by computerized training: Electrophysiological evidence from language-impaired and typically developing children*. Brain Research, 1179, 125-137.
- Stiles, J., & Jernigan, T. L. (2010). The basics of brain development. Neuropsychology Review, 20(4), 327-348.
- Straker, L., Pollock, C., Piek, J., Abbott, R., Skoss, R., Coleman, J., & Leach, R. (2017). Active-input provides more movement and motor skill over passive-input computer gaming. Pediatrics, 139(3), e20161862.
- Sunderland, M. (2007). Helping Children with Fear (Helping Children with Feelings). Speechmark Publishing Ltd.

- Temple, J. R., et al. (2019). The relation between frequency of Facebook use, participation in Facebook activities, and student engagement. Computers & Education, 58(1), 162-171.
- Thomas, A. L., & Johnson, K. L. (2019). An Integrated Approach to Reading Intervention. Journal of Educational Psychology.
- Thomas, A., & Chess, S. (1977). Temperament and Development. Brunner/Mazel.
- Thompson, R. A. (2016). Early attachment and later development: Familiar questions, new answers. In J. Cassidy & P. R. Shaver (Eds.), Handbook of Attachment: Theory, Research, and Clinical Applications (3rd ed., pp. 330-348). Guilford Press.
- Thompson, R. A., & Nelson, C. A. (2001). Developmental science and the media: Early brain development. *American Psychologist, 56*(1), 5-15.
- Trainor, L. J., & Hannon, E. E. (2013). Music acquisition: effects of enculturation and formal training on development. *Trends in Cognitive Sciences, 17*(3), 169-178.
- Tremblay, M. S., LeBlanc, A. G., Kho, M. E., Saunders, T. J., Larouche, R., Colley, R. C., ... & Gorber, S. C. (2011). Systematic review of sedentary behaviour and health indicators in school-aged children and youth. International Journal of Behavioral Nutrition and Physical Activity, 8(1), 98.
- Twenge, J. M., & Campbell, W. K. (2018). Associations between screen time and lower psychological well-being among children and adolescents: Evidence from a population-based study. Preventive Medicine Reports, 12, 271-283.

- Twenge, J. M., Joiner, T. E., Rogers, M. L., & Martin, G. N. (2018). Increases in depressive symptoms, suicide-related outcomes, and suicide rates among U.S. adolescents after 2010 and links to increased new media screen time. Clinical Psychological Science, 6(1), 3-17. DOI: 10.1177/2167702617723376.
- Twenge, J. M., Martin, G. N., & Campbell, W. K. (2018). Decreases in Psychological Well-Being Among American Adolescents After 2012 and Links to Screen Time During the Rise of Smartphone Technology. Emotion, 18(6), 765–780. doi:10.1037/emo0000403
- Uhls, Y. T., et al. (2014). Five days at outdoor education camp without screens improves preteen skills with nonverbal emotion cues. Computers in Human Behavior, 39, 387-392.
- Verburgh, L., Königs, M., Scherder, E. J., & Oosterlaan, J. (2014). Physical exercise and executive functions in preadolescent children, adolescents and young adults: A meta-analysis. British Journal of Sports Medicine, 48(12), 973-979.
- Victora, C. G., Bahl, R., Barros, A. J. D., França, G. V. A., Horton, S., Krasevec, J., ... & Rollins, N. C. (2016). Breastfeeding in the 21st century: epidemiology, mechanisms, and lifelong effect. The Lancet, 387(10017), 475-490.
- Victora, C. G., Bahl, R., Barros, A. J., França, G. V., Horton, S., Krasevec, J., Murch, S., Sankar, M. J., Walker, N., & Rollins, N. C. (2016). Breastfeeding in the 21st century: epidemiology, mechanisms, and lifelong effect. *The Lancet, 387*(10017), 475-490.
- Walker, M. P. (2017). Why we sleep: Unlocking the power of sleep and dreams. Scribner.

- Walker, M. P., & van der Helm, E. (2009). Overnight therapy? The role of sleep in emotional brain function. *Psychological Bulletin*.
- Wartella, E. A., et al. (2016). Parenting in the age of digital technology. Northwestern University.
- Weinstein, A. (2010). Computer and video game addiction—a comparison between game users and non-game users. The American Journal of Drug and Alcohol Abuse, 36(5), 268-276.
- Weisleder, A., & Fernald, A. (2013). Talking to children matters: Early language experience strengthens processing and builds vocabulary. Psychological Science, 24(11), 2143-2152.
- Wentzel, K. R. (2012). Peers and academic functioning at school. *The Oxford Handbook of School Psychology*, 502-513.
- Wolf, M. (2018). Reader, Come Home: The Reading Brain in a Digital World. Harper.
- Wolf, M., Ullman-Shade, C., & Gottwald, S. (2016). How the reading brain resolves the reading paradox: The cognitive circuitry of fluent reading, conversion problems, and why 'in the nick of time' interventions challenge the whole child. *Developmental Medicine & Child Neurology*, 58(S4), 25-34.
- Zenner, C., Herrnleben-Kurz, S., & Walach, H. (2014). Mindfulness-based interventions in schools—A systematic review and meta-analysis. *Frontiers in Psychology, 5*, 603. https://doi.org/10.3389/fpsyg.2014.00603
- Zimmerman, F. J., Christakis, D. A., & Meltzoff, A. N. (2007). Television and DVD/video viewing in children younger than 2 years. Archives of Pediatrics & Adolescent Medicine, 161(5), 473-479. DOI: 10.1001/archpedi.161.5.473.

- Zunshine, L. (2021). The Cultural Evolution of Fictional Empathy. Linguistic Inquiry, 52(1), 1-36.

www.ingramcontent.com/pod-product-compliance
Lightning Source LLC
Chambersburg PA
CBHW062048270326
41931CB00013B/2986
* 9 7 9 8 9 9 2 5 4 8 2 2 8 *